COSETTE HAUGEN

Sockfoot Soldier

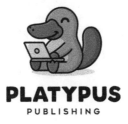

PLATYPUS
PUBLISHING

To Than, of course

Acknowledgement

Writing this book felt like doing physical therapy after an injury. I knew it was necessary for my long term well-being, but actually doing it ranged from minor annoyance to downright pain. Having to reopen the wounds and immerse myself back into those feelings was not easy. So I want to recognize two groups of people: the ones who helped me turn this trauma into a literary achievement, and the ones who got me through the trauma in the first place.

The two groups overlap *a lot*.

Let me start by thanking those who helped turn the story into the book you are about to read. These people remind me of a good crossword puzzle—fantastic to spend a Sunday with over coffee, and always teaching me something new.

To Jen Lakin, Kavya Johnson, Alex Panayiotou for their early encouragement and thoughtful reviews. And Ishmam Ahmed for all that plus masterminding any particular sentence or metaphor that I just could not make work.

To Adam Marcotte, Heidi Haugen, Yena Lee, Faroz Mujir, Laura Paolino, and Heidi Liedtke for being cheerleaders to the marathon of this book's development.

To Matt Rudnitsky for the advice and answers on how to write a book, to Des Tan for giving a damn, and to Hannah Klein for the polishing, perfecting, and perspective.

To Ashley Cardona for the lessons on explication, which

taught me how to discern meaning from poetry and thus began the lesson of how to do the same for life.

And to Eric Tank for graciously permitting me to include Lauren in this story.

Then, I want to acknowledge the big supporters, especially those from around that June and the months that followed. This collection of people remind me of good New Yorker cartoons—clever, relatable, witty, and worth putting pictures of on my refrigerator to make me grin.

To the random guy who helped me on the bridge and made sure I was in good hands and to my fellow "inmates" of the ward who made the stay tolerable and certainly memorable. I am especially thankful for those of you still in my life.

To everyone who visited and made all the difference in the world by being there.

To my team at Accenture who did everything right and helped make the rest of my recovery smooth.

To Brenton Cozby, Valkyrie Jensen and Tiffany Luong for leaping up to help me celebrate this book's publication on time and in style.

To Grace Pyo, Antonina Malyarenko, Nara Paulsen, Molly Owens, and Katrina Rudisel for the post-hospitalization friendship and kindness, and to Sabrina Bias who transformed me into a rainbow and helped me match my appearance to how my soul wanted to feel.

And to Pigeon the cat for keeping my lap warm as I wrote.

Finally, it goes without saying that there is an entire crowd of friends, family members, colleagues, mentors, artists, public figures, kind strangers, and other cuddly animals that I would also like to thank for this gift of a life.

I

Reconnaissance

1

Big Girls Cry

The woman is huddled on the corridor floor, folded into herself, with her knees to her chest. Nurses and counselors are walking by without a second look. The woman's mewling whimpers are coldly disregarded. The psych ward does not halt for anyone's misery.

From my doorway, the woman is directly across from me. I have not seen her before—she must be one of the patients who always sleep and never leave their rooms. Why is no one tending to her?

One counselor finally glances down on his way past. He barely registers the woman's cries. He keeps walking. Does he think she is just acting this way "for attention"?

Does it matter?

Hearing her makes my heart ache, but I am in no state to be comforting anyone. I would not be able to muster up a single word of hope or consolation to her. So I am useless too.

Down the hall, Billie is talking exuberantly to someone on the mobile phone. Her resonant voice echoes. "They call me Red—or Mama bear," she says. "It's hysterical. It's—*oh honey.*"

Billie has noticed the crying woman and drops the phone to hurry over. She bends down deeply to look the woman in the eyes.

"Shh, baby," Billie whispers. "Baby, you can't let them see you cry."

I cannot hear the woman's mumbling response, but she is gripping Billie's outstretched hands like they are a lifeline.

"Can I get you some water?" Billie asks. "Or do you want something to calm you down? I bet I could get you an Ativan, if you want one."

Again, I cannot hear the woman's mumbles, but she must have said yes because Billie yells at the counselor on duty.

"Can you get this poor woman a glass of water?"

The counselor just blinks unresponsively. The drinking fountain is five feet from his station and even has a stack of paper cups, but he does not move.

"Come on, get up and help!" Billie yells, frustrated. "Can't you people do anything *kind*?"

"I can't leave my post," the counselor replies.

"For the love of God, what is wrong with you? You were just going to sit there and do nothing while this woman is clearing suffering and in pain. You should be ashamed." Billie starts to unwrap her hands from the woman's grip, but the woman holds tight.

Just as Billie is about to yell to the counselor again, I emerge from my doorway and grab a cup from the stack. I fill it with water. It only takes three seconds.

Not making eye contact with the guard, Billie, or the woman, I placed the paper cup down next to them on the floor and start shuffling over to the nurse's station.

"Thank you, sweetie," Billie calls after me.

I reach the nurse's station and tap on the window. A nurse answers my knock.

"There's a woman down there who I think might want an Ativan to calm down," I mumble quietly.

"Okay," The nurse says. "Do you know who?"

"I don't know her name. Billie's with her."

"'Kay. An Ativan, you said?"

"Yeah," I reply. "And I'll take one too."

2

The Fall Into Presence

The Bloomingdale Line in northern Chicago was once a 2.7-mile elevated railroad that has since been converted into green space as part of the 606 park and trail system. It extends eastward, allowing foot and bicycle traffic to cross over dozens of north-south streets and nearly reach Lake Michigan. For me, a twenty-three-year-old transplant from Minneapolis who was used to having access to marshland pathways, the 606 was a haven. I had been living in Logan Square for almost a year but, for a multitude of reasons, it still did not feel like home.

Except on the 606.

There, people were at their neighborly best. Legging-clad women walking in pairs, gaggles of children skipping ahead of their parents, young professionals walking their new puppies—everyone seemed happy. And when I was on the 606, fueled by endorphins and vitamin D, bicycling with the best friends I had the privilege of calling my roommates, I usually felt happy too.

Tonight started that way.

It was unusual for me to be out and about on a weekday. As a consultant, I worked Monday through Thursday of most weeks in a different city. On a normal Thursday, I would have flown from the client site back home to Chicago that day, arrived at O'Hare by 6:00 p.m., said hello to whichever of my two roommates was home by 7:00 p.m. and crawled into bed for the rest of the evening. This week, I had returned home a day early—work had been especially demanding—and I conducted all of my meetings from our sunlit living room. So I said yes when my roommate, Than, had popped his head over my laptop to ask if I wanted to catch an improv show. For once, on a Thursday, it felt like I had the energy.

We rode our bikes to the iO theater, where the improv troupes Smokin' Hot Dads and Meridian did an admirable job of helping me forget the past three days' stress. When we had started riding back on the 606, well past dusk, I told Than to go on ahead and that I would I meet him back home. He needed to bike at the pace of a guy who had a long-distance girlfriend to devotedly call and I wanted to enjoy the nighttime June air.

Almost no one else was on the trail this evening. Since there was no traffic and the breeze was sweet, I unbuckled my helmet, slung it over my handlebars, and let my hair fly behind me. It was lovely outside, and I had nowhere else I needed to be but present.

And yet—of course! Of course, just when I was starting to approach clarity and appreciate the evening peace of the 606, that familiar coldness washed over me. My mind started running, the black sky started sinking and suddenly my joints felt stiff and my gut tight. Ahead, I saw that bench.

I let my bicycle clatter to the pavement and sat so that I was overlooking Campbell Street. The air that had just been so sweet turned noxious. I could barely breathe. I wrapped my arms around my body to keep myself intact. I tried to breathe slowly but felt the pressure build behind my eyelids.

Even though death was nowhere near, it felt like it was everywhere.

But I did not want to die.

While I sat, a small number of nighthawks passed behind me on skates, boards, bicycles, or their sneakers. Big fat defeated tears started to trickle down my face, sprouting from those intrusive thoughts about the pace of life and the weight of its inherent sadness and unfairness. All of that ache, spilling from my eyeballs on the 606. And despite the street lamps, no one noticed me.

I knew there were two big reasons no one stopped to ask if I was okay. One was practical—my hunched back was turned away from the path; unless they looked closely, no one could see my face. And even if they did, there was reason number two—public courtesy conditions most people to Not Disturb the Crying Stranger.

But it felt like all of Chicago was actively ignoring my pain. And so even though I was in love with the city for a hundred different reasons, at that moment I hated it.

I broke apart, heaving soundlessly. I called all the numbers of people I knew within a mile radius but was met mostly with overly cheerful greetings and leave-a-message-at-the-beeps. A few friends answered, but I found I did not know what to say. So I said "hello", then said "okay bye," and returned to crying. I began to spiral so inwardly that I forgot how to speak.

At least thirty minutes of silent sobbing passed before someone even came into my vicinity. The guy was tall and had a sharp jaw and bulging backpack. Wisely, he sat a safe distance away on a different bench, hesitant to move closer until he could assess my mental state (which was not good, in case that was not clear by now).

Over another half an hour, he inched closer. In between my silent pleas to an unresponsive heaven and broken sobs into my knees, I had been trying to make eye contact with him. Finally, he stood up and walked the last few yards.

"You good?"

I shook my head.

"You diabetic or something?"

And I shook my head more slowly, moving my bag and phone to the ground, hoping he would sit next to me, but he kept a wide berth between us.

"Can I call someone for you?" he tried again.

My words were trapped safely in my throat where they could not turn into screams, so as an answer, I handed him the card of a psychologist I once saw that I keep in my wallet. It has written on it, *To emergency personnel, please call this number.* With my finger, I traced the emergency telephone number on the bench between us. He understood enough to start digging for a pen in his backpack.

"I've only got this," he said, holding out a blue Sharpie and uncapping it for me.

I wrote *9-1-1* in wobbly letters right on the bench. The marker was fresh and each line bled instantly into the wood grain. As the man leapt up to try and flag someone else down, I kept writing. *Need help. Mental Health. Please call.*

"Do you have a phone?" I heard the man shout to someone. "She needs help! We need to call an ambulance!"

He had managed to wave down a 606 bike patroller who skidded to a stop but would not hand over his phone out of suspicion.

"You don't have a phone?" the patroller asked the guy. He probably thought we were pulling something.

"She needs help! She's diabetic or something, I just need to call!"

No, I thought. Not diabetic. Depressed. Scared. Frozen. In danger.

I held out my phone in my limp hand and motioned toward the two of them while they continued to go back and forth about diabetes. The patroller finally noticed the phone and dialed, talking first to the operator, trying to explain where we were, what was going on, and leaving out all the important information that I had scribbled on the bench and was hitting with my palm.

Halfway through the patroller's frenzied phone call, the two of them exchanged names. The first man, Hector, explained that he and I did not know each other but that he had just stopped to help. The patroller, who had an unmemorable name like Josh or John, kept rubbing my back as I held my knees and rocked back and forth.

I knew I was being taken care of and I let myself float away into a semi-conscious state.

I remember Patroller Josh or John racing to the nearest 606 on-ramp to escort the paramedics over.

I remember walking like a zombie over to the bike rack to lock up my bicycle while Hector hovered around me trying to help.

I remember being strapped unnecessarily to the paramedics' gurney and then being wheeled into the back of the ambulance.

I remember nodding and shaking at the paramedics' questions. For some questions, I typed the answer on my phone and then turned the screen to one paramedic—the nice, bald, middle-aged one, not the short Latina one who kept insisting, "She can talk, she just doesn't *want* to."

I remember relaying that I was taking two hundred milligrams daily of my antidepressant, sertraline; no, I had not taken anything else; and no, I did not have a plan to hurt myself.

I remember zipping through Bucktown, Wicker Park, and Westtown, sirens blaring.

I remember being wheeled into the ER and escorted toward the back while the front desk clerk commented, "Another one, huh?"

I remember passing my phone, ID, insurance card, and bicycle helmet to a kindly ER nurse with teal scrubs. I remember loopily signing some "Received for Care" document with two letters of my signature and getting a scannable wristband with my name and DOB.

I remember changing into a blue paper gown and blue paper shorts in a bathroom with only a swinging shoulder-height mat for a door.

I remember how my room in the back corner of the ER smelled like urine. I remember the grunting snores of the few homeless men sleeping something off for the night.

I remember waiting, waiting, waiting, for someone to tell me what happened now.

I remember crying more, silently at first, but then loudly and desperately, for *someone* to pay me a bit of attention.

When I came back fully aware and lucid, I had not spoken to another soul for what must have been an hour. But now, with the front of my paper gown soaked with hot tears, I had the full and presuming attention of a doctor named Dr. Patel.

He introduced himself, confirmed my date of birth, and dove right in.

"So you want to kill yourself, hmm?"

3

Controlled Catatonia

I have been clinically depressed for all of my adult life and—call it morbid fascination—the idea of suicide has always intrigued me. From what I have felt firsthand and then later read about to try and understand, I believe there are two characteristics that, if simultaneously present, could make anyone want to kill themselves.

Everybody experiences pain throughout their life. It is part of being human. And, as the self-deprecating and often self-pitying creatures that we are, many of us also at some point or another consider that the world would be better off without us.

Now, my theory goes that if (A) a person is in an intense amount of pain, and (B) they believe with every ounce of their being that the world could be better without them in it, then yes, that person will want to die. And if the circumstances are right, they will be willing to die by their own hand.

Both of those things must be true, but the kicker is that it makes no difference how *long* they are true—just that they happen simultaneously. It could be for a split second. But if that second is in front of a train, at a busy street, or with a loaded gun in hand, then it's Game Over.

I am no stranger to the pain—physical or psychological. Chronic migraines, constant aches, mental anguish from anxiety, or general fatigue from depression—it is all painful. So when I can feel those The-World-Would-Be-Better-Off-Without-You Blues, I use caution. I find my loved ones. I avoid alcohol and intersections.

And pain distorts reality. Pain amplifies isolation. It sniggers into our ears that we do not matter. It steals our rationality and returns us to a state of child logic where emotion hijacks our good sense and impairs our judgment. Pain driving negative behavior is easier to identify in contained occasions, in single outbursts. It is harder to spot in a drawn-out depressive episode. Having to constantly remind yourself that the pain is worth it, that people cherish you, is exhausting.

That night in June, I was exhausted.

But I did not want to kill myself.

I did not want to die.

So to answer Dr. Patel's question, I shook my head no.

"You want to hurt yourself?" he tried again, staring down at whatever was on his handheld screen.

I shook my head no again.

"You know you can talk. No one is going to hurt you."

But that was not correct—I was here because I was scared *I* would hurt myself. Not that I wanted to. That's why I was here—to *not* hurt myself.

"They told me you said you were suicidal. Is that true?"

I wracked my brain for what I might have nodded or shaken my head at when the paramedics were asking me questions. I must have taken too long to respond though, because Dr. Patel moved on with, "That's okay, it was good to come here."

Later I found out that he had written *Suicidal inclination* in my chart, even though that was a massive bastardization of what I had typed out on a note page on my phone. Once I was discharged, I looked back in my phone's notes and saw fragments typed out. Nowhere did it allude to killing or suicide or death.

Dr. Patel continued to ask questions and answer them himself. I never made eye contact because if I looked directly at him, I felt I might—I don't know—spontaneously combust. I wished he would have asked clearer yes-or-no questions, or at least paused a minute to let me whisper out words, but everything I wanted to say kept getting caught in my throat. I wanted him to know that at that moment I was preoccupied and concentrating on not dying, not screaming, not bolting out the door, not letting myself jump in front of an oncoming ambulance or grabbing *that* syringe off *that* med cart or shoving *that* instrument into the wall socket *right there*.

He was evaluating an incoming patient but I was on impulse control. At the moment, my objective was more important.

Dr. Patel finally left without providing me any answers or an indication of how long he would be gone or where I would be escorted to next. From my curled position on the hard plastic bench, I waited.

At some point, another nurse came in to take vials of my blood—she did not say why—and it was another lifetime of waiting until a different ER nurse who saw my distorted look of agony rushed to give me "something to calm you down, sweetie," which meant an Ativan and a cup of ice water.

"How long...here?" I asked brokenly, motioning to the 10x10 room I was being held in. Even though there was a more comfortable-looking gurney across the room, I was using the bench as a makeshift bed because I did not want to be near the stretcher's mess of metallic bars and binding straps.

"They're looking to find a bed for you upstairs. Dr. Patel didn't tell you?"

Headshake.

"I don't know how long it'll be though, hon," the nurse said. "How about I turn these blinds down and close the door a bit and you can try to get some sleep."

It was a statement, not a question, and I resigned myself to lying down on the plastic, using the blanket as a pillow and covering myself as best as I could in my paper gown. The nurse brought me another blanket and I closed my eyes, trying to ignore the snores and smells of other patients outside my door.

I had been in an ER waiting area once before, for a similar reason. In the late fall of my freshman year of college, I had experienced a mental health breakdown much like this one. My friends, two of whom were the same men I lived with now, had been relaxing in my dorm room when they realized I had been gone for quite a while and opened the door to find me puddled in a teary-eyed heap against the stairwell threshold.

"9-1-1," I had said to my friends, clutching my arms.

They stayed with me until a police officer arrived. The officer put me in the back seat of his squad car and we drove from the Honors Dorm to the hospital three blocks away.

It was late in the evening that time too, and I spent hours and hours perched on a gurney with a different officer stationed outside my room. I was not allowed to sleep—I could not even turn off the lights. I remember watching *CSI: Miami* reruns until 6:00 a.m. and trying to be friendly to the cop by asking if he wanted to watch too since he had to stay awake anyway.

16

At least this time around, I was allowed to try and rest.

I do not know what time it was when Dr. Patel finally woke me from whatever daze or state of sleep I was in. He told me they had a room on the fifteenth floor. I did not know what that meant, but I followed him meekly through another maze of hallways, into an elevator, and out onto a brightly lit landing where I was passed off to somebody else whose name might have been Jean. I never saw Dr. Patel again and to this day, I would not be able to pick him out from a line-up. He might have had short hair?

Maybe-Jean weighed me, took my blood pressure, took five more vials of blood, gave me blue scrub pants, a hospital gown, mesh underwear, and two pairs of hospital socks (one light brown, one baby blue). She checked my body for signs of self-harm and asked me how I was feeling ("Really tired"). Somebody else handed me a brown paper bag, the type I used to pack a lunch in, with toiletries inside. Without any other word of information, I was led to room 1525 and told I could sleep, but to always keep the door ajar so they could do bed checks.

I did not look around the room much, just noticed that I had my own bathroom with a curtain for a door and that the bed was bolted to the floor but not up against the wall. My mind had no capacity to think or overthink. I changed out of my paper clothes and into the hospital ones, then climbed in between the stiff sheets, under the two thin blankets, and finally—*finally*—slept.

❮ iCloud

June 8, 2017 at 11:54 PM

My address

My SSN

200 mg sertraline daily

I need to keep these thoughts in my head until I can give them to a shrink

One at apartment is his birthday, I don't want to bother him

Wasn't trying, just fixating

Wanted to so didn't move
Hector was sitting next to me for a long time

Old ID, just moved in August

Anxiety (GAD) OCD according to some docs

Not for the past two months

I want to be here

I feel out of control
I don't want to talk
Not particularly
Lebanon Greece
May 11 got back may 29

Not anymore
Lots of people
Minnesota
Was only in California for <1 year
MN is home
1 year

Maybe to sleep but not now
I feel hyper calm

Where am I?

4

This Is Normal

The Wilhelm Scream is a frequently-used sound effect that has been featured in nearly four hundred movies and numerous TV episodes. Sheb Wooley is the voice actor credited with it after it was first used in the 1951 film *Distant Drums*. I guarantee you have heard it before—it is that high-pitched, blood-curdling scream that plays when characters are thrown off buildings, surprised by the horrible monster, or shot. And it's almost exactly the sound I woke up to that first morning in the ward.

The hell?!

I might have jolted out of bed if I had not been so dazed. My overtired brain took a moment to acknowledge my unfamiliar surroundings before I kicked the sheets off of my clammy feet and shuffled to my doorway.

A small group of timid hospital-gowned women was watching something around the corner. The screaming morphed to yelling ("Get off of me! Let me out!") but no one seemed terribly concerned so I did not bother investigating further. Maybe this was just how things were.

I found a clock on the wall outside my room. It was well

before 7:00 a.m. There was a staff member, who I later learned was called a "counselor," sitting in a chair below the clock. She gave me a look that clearly said, *don't worry about the yelling.* So I didn't worry about the yelling.

When you think about it, there are not too many occasions for adults to really scream. I am referring to the clear, piercing, depths-of-your-being type of shrieks, like the ones I had just heard. Besides roller coasters and the occasional dark prank, adults do not have too many opportunities to let their vocal cords go.

But here in the ward—at the butt-crack of dawn, no less—someone had already found that opportunity.

This turned out to be a regular occurrence, but the first time was jarring. My general tiredness and prior night's Ativan kept me from being *too* jarred, but still, heart palpitations were not my preferred method of morning arousal.

My thoughts and feelings were back in my control even though only a few hours had passed since my admittance. I was still feeling tired and heavy, but I had been feeling that way for months. If I had woken up in my own bed instead of on this hospital cot, I would have made coffee and booted up my computer like I would on any other day.

Sitting on my bed, I could take proper stock of my room for the first time. Overall, it was bare and beige. The only piece of furniture was the bed—no side table even. The room's fluorescent light was caged in and at eye height against the wall nearest (but not touching!) the bed. To the left of the door were two empty grocery-sized paper bags with the handles removed, for trash, and a shabby storage unit painted orange with two low open shelves on one side and a locked cabinet door on the other.

Opposite the door-and-storage wall was a narrow window with a vent at the base, opening to a western view of Chicago and all its rectangular homes. The dusty linoleum was beige, like the walls, like the tarp-like curtain, and the would-be electrical sockets were covered with metal panels. There were no hooks, very few edges and no decor.

During the night, someone had placed another paper bag with my name on it on one of the shelves, and I peered inside to find all my street clothes from the night before, except for my bra.

I peeked into the bathroom, which I had all but ignored in my hurry to fall asleep the night before. Now, behind the curtain, I saw a low toilet with its tank tucked away into the wall, a commercial-looking sink, and a shower that reminded me of the community swimming pool showers rooms by its damp smell and brown tiles. I noticed a box above the toilet that read, *Pull string to call nurse*, only the string had been removed.

Emptying the contents of my complimentary toiletry bag, I lined up the hypoallergenic two-in-one shampoo and body wash, hypoallergenic lotion, packets of toothpaste, a flimsy white toothbrush, wrapped bar soap, a white tube of Vaseline and roll-on deodorant against the mirror. I noticed that some patient before me had etched a hundred lines into the glass with who-knows-what. I used the toilet, trying to make the curtain close as tightly as possible, and then washed my hands with the thin bar of soap. When I stepped out, another "counselor" was standing with a blood pressure machine and saying my name.

"Looks normal," he said at my usual 120ish over 80ish.

I asked if I was going to talk to a psychiatrist or a therapist soon.

"Probably," he said. "After breakfast."

He did not know any more specific details.

"When's breakfast?"

"Later. Maybe 8:30 p.m." And he continued onto the next room.

I noticed the same patients had passed by my room a few times, doing laps around the ward. After putting on my light blue hospital socks and tee shirt from the night before, I ventured out and started an exploratory lap myself.

The entire ward hallway made a square, with all the thirty or so identical patient room doorways on the outer wall so each room could have a window to the Outside. Surrounded by the ward, on the other side of the inner hallway walls, there was the elevator bank that had brought me up, an administrative desk and, if I remember correctly, some offices, but it was completely inaccessible to us, thanks to a heavy locked door.

My room, 1525, was near the northwest corner of the floor and right across from the drinking fountain, which miraculously gushed ice-cold water. At both the northwest and southeast corners sat stationed counselors who had full views of their respective hallways so that all activity, at all times, could be monitored. Also at the southeast corner and barred to us was the nurse's station, with its three windows that you had to tap repeatedly to get a nurse's attention since their backs were always turned to face the windows and the Chicago skyline. Next to the nurse's station was Dayroom B, with the piano and the functioning TV, and, across the hall on the inner ring, was the exam room and the contraband closet. The northeast corner housed Dayroom A and had patient-made art on the walls. The hallway was peppered with posters that said things like *Keep Calm and Ask.* The daily schedule, which I eventually learned was a complete farce, was posted in each dayroom and across from the nurse's station. Signs with resident rights and phone hours were posted around as well.

On my second or third lap, a woman started keeping pace next to me. She had salt-and-pepper hair almost to her shoulders, a concerned-looking red face and was wearing hospital pants and an orange shirt with purple and teal tassels.

"You're new," she stated matter-of-factly. "I'm Billie. I'm so sorry you're in here."

My throat felt scratchy and I still had not brushed my teeth, so I responded with a limp, "Yeah, thanks," and kept walking.

She continued to walk beside me, saying nothing, and I was too listless to protest.

The few laps we walked together in silence gave my mind a chance to regroup. Walking is great for thinking productively.

Last night I had felt out of control, like I had been walking on some precipice without somewhere safe to jump down to. I no longer felt that way—time and sleep always help—but I still felt exhausted. I knew the out-of-control-and-overwhelmed-and-about-to-die feeling was just below the surface. Anything could make it erupt and then it would just be another cascade like last night.

I don't need *to be here anymore*, I thought. *But if they can help, then why not stay and see?*

This "decision" to stay was just an illusion of choice. But I did not know that yet.

As Billie and I rounded another corner, I could feel my nose start to bleed. I excused myself from our partnered walk ("See ya later, I guess...") to tend to my bloody nose.

No Kleenex in the bathrooms. And I wasn't about to put single-ply toilet paper up my nostril just to have it disintegrate into a literal bloody pulp. I turned on the cold sink tap, covered up the other nostril and just blew. Each droplet made a firework in the sink and then bled toward the drain. I blew harder until the blood clot came out and then rubbed down the sink until there were no traces of pink left. After wiping my face, I looked back up to inspect the remaining damage in the mirror.

Fuck, I looked awful. After barely any sleep, my usual under-eye bags had doubled so that there were now *two* heavy lines under each eye. There was redness, oiliness, and I was still an uneven shade tanner from my last vacation. Things needed to be popped and plucked. And my hair was still in some semblance of a bun, meaning I could see every bit of my face and I hated what I saw.

Turning away in disgust, I flopped back onto my bed to stare at my ceiling and kept staring for over an hour until I heard a heavy cart roll past my door.

Someone called out, "Breakfast, ladies!"

I was not hungry, but I *was* bored.

I wandered out of my room in my sock-feet and stayed near the back of the small group gathering around the tall silver food cart. I had only seen a handful of other patients on my morning laps with Billie, but now I saw around a dozen. We were women of all ages, races and states of unkemptness. I hugged myself, thinking that I certainly looked the part.

We each had a tray assigned to us, denoted by a flimsy receipt with our name, room number, and whether we were "vegetarian" or "regular." My tray was handed to me and I followed the other women to Dayroom A. Only half of the women ate in here—for crowd control, I suppose. The other side of the ward got their food from a second silver cart and ate in Dayroom B. A handful were permitted to eat in their own rooms.

There were three smaller square tables around the dayroom and a long rectangular one in the middle. Billie motioned for me to sit next to her at the long one and she announced to everyone that I was new.

"I'm Nina," said a woman with dyed red hair, premature wrinkles and a radiant smile. "Just so you know, the food tastes like ass."

"I'm Angelique," said a much younger and larger Latina woman with glasses.

"And that's Delilah," Billie pointed to a massive slack-jawed woman with stubble at the head of the table who would not talk all day, "and Brenda," —another large, slack-jawed woman with dyed red hair who slurred hello, "and Francine."

"I'm Francine," said Francine. She looked older than she probably was, had shiny dark brown skin, and sat in a wheelchair. Like Delilah and Brenda, she was wearing two hospital gowns, one tied forward, one tied backward, whereas Nina, Angelique and Billie were wearing a mashup of their street clothes plus hospital garb.

"We didn't get your name, sweetie," said Nina.

I told them.

"That's a nice name," Francine slurred, spoon halfway to her mouth.

"It is a nice name, isn't it, Francine?" Billie validated.

I looked down at my tray and saw a sad scoop of eggs, dried out French toast sticks, a fruit cup and a black plastic coffee mug kept "warm" by a clear plastic lid. I wanted none of it but nibbled at some pale pineapple while the ladies gave me the run of the place.

"Yeah, the food's always shit but you gotta eat it or else you'll just be starvin'," Nina explained. "And the coffee's decaf and it's never hot, but sometimes it's pretty warm."

"And save your hot chocolate packets 'cause you can get hot water out of your sink and drink it later," Billie advised.

"I didn't get hot chocolate," I said, noticing for the first time that every person's breakfast was slightly different.

"Yeah, you can choose it on your menu," Nina said, showing me how she was already circling items on hers with a crayon. "You'll get one tomorrow and then you can get better stuff than the automatic tray—not that any of it's good."

Brenda let out a startling "ha!" from the opposite end of the table, causing her to miss her mouth with her bagel and ending up with a smear of cream cheese on her cheek.

"I guess that was funny," Nina said, shrugging with a grin.

I liked Nina instantly. Her voice was warm and gravelly, and her eyes smiled even when her mouth chewed.

A girl my age with short rockabilly black bangs and a septum piercing shuffled in looking pale and tired. We made room for her at our table. She introduced herself as Mia and told us she had been admitted the night before, same as me, after her friends convinced her she needed to hospitalize herself.

I looked Mia up and down and compared myself to her. Getting admitted at the same time makes you something like twins at the psych ward. It starts an unspoken race over who can get released first.

Breakfast did not last long and I mostly listened—or tried to. My ability to concentrate did not feel up to scratch, but I managed to learn a bit about everyone at the table. Nina had granddaughters, Billie had a benign brain tumor that made her deaf in her right ear and fucked up half of her facial nerves, and

27

Brenda was on a high dose of Effexor that day and was currently one of three Brenda's on the ward. (Old Brenda, straight out of a nursing home, was sitting at one of the smaller tables and getting out that day, and Little Brenda mostly kept to herself.)

When we had stomached all we could, the trays went back in the silver cart and we returned to our rooms. I went back to staring at the ceiling and tried not to keep at bay all the questions swirling in my head. Really, it was just one question in different forms: *Now what?*

It was not long before there was a knock on my open door and a plainly dressed woman with nice hair peered in. The badge around her neck identified her as a nurse practitioner, which I knew meant that she could prescribe me medication; I had seen an NP all throughout college on a semi-regular basis to fill my sertraline prescription.

"I'm Mackenzie," the NP said, not extending her hand. "How are you feeling?"

I told her I was fine, just tired, and said that she was welcome to sit at the edge of my bed.

She declined and continued, "So you've been feeling depressed, and have had thoughts of suicide?"

I bobbed my head side to side and clarified, "Definitely depressed, but I haven't been suicidal. I told the ER doctor last night—it's just like I can't get these thoughts of death out of my head."

"What do you mean?"

"I mean, I look at everything and just see how it could kill me. Or I look at people and think about how their lives could keep going on without me. But I don't want to die. And I don't want to hurt myself. I love the people in my life way too much for that."

28

She jotted things down as I spoke, then said, "How's your medication been working for you?"

"Honestly," I said, "not great. I know I'm maxed out on sertraline and I've been feeling pretty depressed and fatigued for the past three months."

"Yeah," Mackenzie said, still looking down at her chart. "We can't prescribe any more than two hundred milligrams for an adult."

"I know."

"We can switch you to something else?"

"That sounds good," I answered, expecting that would be the case. It had crossed my mind a few times over the past six months, but I had never gotten the ball rolling. Changing meds is a real bitch.

Mackenzie continued, "Has anything happened in your life to trigger this episode?"

"Episode—like last night?"

"Like, this depressive episode."

"Oh."

And so I gave her the synopsis—the suicides and attempted suicides of friends far too young and much too loved; the pressure at work followed by the departure of an incredible manager; the difficulty of adjusting to a new city; the stagnant love life; the ex that had just gotten engaged; and the news that one of my best-friend-roommates had just accepted a job across the country.

"But really," I said evenly, "I think I could normally handle all that if I didn't feel so goddamn lonely."

"Hmm," Mackenzie said. "That's a lot."

"Life is a lot."

"Well, it's good that you're here. Is there anyone I can notify for you?"

Since my phone, bike helmet, purse, and all other belongings had been confiscated, I nodded yes with as much vigor as I could muster. If Than had realized I had not come home last night, I knew he would be very worried. And my manager needed to know why I would not be online.

"You can tell them both that I'm here, in the psych ward—I don't care. It won't be *too* much of a surprise," I added. "They know I'm depressed. I'm pretty open about this stuff."

"I'll tell them," Mackenzie said. "Do you know their numbers?"

"You'll have to look them up on my phone," I explained, and I gave her the contact names.

She told me she would contact them and left to move on to the next patient's room. Our conversation could not have lasted more than ten minutes. As far as I am aware, she was the only person with discharging abilities to visit the whole ward that day, and I wish I had been told that she had the same privileges as a psychiatrist. Technically, she never told me what her responsibilities were. I only knew she was an NP because I saw her badge. If I had known, I would have told her so much more.

No doctor came in the next day either. I would not talk to anyone with prescribing or discharging privileges until fifty-three hours later. Weekends in the ward were like Gotham—vigilante justice ruled the day.

5

A Good Handshake

No one likes being the new kid. Whether it is a new school or a new workplace—even a new fitness class—every moment is steeped in hyperawareness. Suddenly you are thinking about everything you are doing, including what you say, how you say it, how you hold your hands—the fact that you *have* hands that you need to do something with. It feels like everyone is sizing you up and putting you into a box, even though the more logical part of you knows most people are not giving you a second thought. Still, you are on high alert and on the lookout for opportunities to be clever or leave a good impression. Every move matters and you get exhausted from overthinking.

That is how I felt those first few hours on the fifteenth floor, but times five. And the stakes were higher. Stand out, and I risked being ostracized by other crazy people, or even worse, misjudged by those who could grant me freedom.

So much depends upon
a red-faced patient
glazed with perspiration
beside the white-haired women

All of the impression-forming and bonding happened in the dayrooms. Haphazardly throughout the day, sessions that the schedule referred to as "therapy" took place here too. There were never any announcements that therapy was occurring. The first morning, I only found out that there was an "art therapy" session happening after wandering absentmindedly to Dayroom A where I found a motley crew of patients lazily coloring in prints of butterflies and flowers or digging through a giant bucket of plastic beads.

I balked. This hour-long access to crayons, markers, and paper did not constitute art therapy. It was barely arts and crafts.

True art therapy is a fairly controversial form of healing in the psychology world. It's *supposed* to be a form of expressive therapy that uses the process of creating art to improve a person's well-being. Basically, the thinking is that if you can express yourself artistically, you can use that to resolve internalized issues and learn to manage feelings, improve self-esteem, increase personal awareness, reduce stress—all that jazz. Its merit and effectiveness are argued pretty heavily, as I understand, because there are lots of ways to do it *in*effectively. But it is one of the more common forms of group therapy because it is mostly nonverbal, easy to facilitate, and cheap.

I saw Nina, Angelique, red-haired Big Brenda, Francine, and Billie at the big center table, along with a happy-faced woman with crooked teeth and short hair dyed highlighter yellow. Delilah, as drugged as ever, was at a smaller table with a Filipina woman named Little Brenda and a wispy-haired Latina woman named Carla who rarely spoke.

The session was overseen by Fiona, a wideset sandy-haired counselor in her fifties whose light blue polo stretched obscenely across her chest. She gave a hello and flurried her hand at the craft cart she guarded.

"Take anything you'd like," she said sunnily.

I dug through the stack of goofy, childish prints and pulled out a picture of a giraffe and a coconut tree. Grabbing a few crayons and a set of watercolor paints, I sat at the long table and settled in.

Most of the women were beading; someone mentioned that today was the first time they had actual string to make necklaces and bracelets. Fiona had sprung for a spool of plasticky orange string, like the kind you make keychains out of at summer camp. I was pretty sure the plastic string constituted a safety hazard—I remembered my sneakers had not been returned to me. Apparently, you could choke somebody with shoelaces or hang yourself with a bra, but a long spool of plastic floss was perfectly innocuous.

I got to work drawing waxy brown lines on my palm tree while Billie sidled up to me again.

"How are you doing?" she asked, and I told her I was fine—still not feeling chatty—but she kept on. "Look at these pretty beads. Aren't they nice?"

"Check out these ones I've got," the highlighter-haired girl said. Then she turned to me to introduce herself. "I'm Patty. Who're you?"

"Cosette," I said, adding yellow swirls to my giraffe.

"She got here last night," Nina added. "Mia too. Where's Mia? She napping?"

"Yup," said Billie. "She probably needs it. And it's her first day so she doesn't need to get group points too bad yet."

"Group points?" I asked.

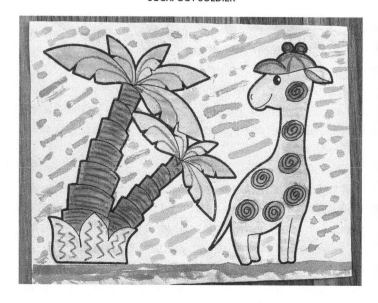

"Yeah," Nina said. "They take attendance when we go to group. And if you go to group more, you get out sooner 'cause they keep track, see. Angelique, can you help me tie this like you tied yours?" She handed her long chain of white, pink, and blue beads to Angelique, who apparently was the best at tying the slippery string.

"That's beautiful," Fiona was saying to someone at another table.

"Brenda, wake up!"

Big Brenda, nodding off and drooling, was shaken awake by Billie. "Wha—?"

"You were falling asleep again, hon," Nina explained. "Damn, they got you *drugged up*!"

"You can't let them do that to you, Brenda," Billie added. "You've got to advocate for yourself! And ask them what the side effects are before you take anything. They wanted to give me *lithium* and that's a contraindication for cancer and I have a *brain tumor.*"

Big Brenda made a noise and went back to coloring in her picture, only to nod off again a few minutes later.

Angelique finished tying up Nina's chain and handed it back to her. "Would it look dumb if I put it on my head?" Nina asked, demonstrating.

"I like it," Patty said.

"It looks like a flower crown," I commented truthfully. "Like you're going to a music festival. I also thought it made her look like she belonged in a psych ward, but I kept that to myself. The longer I looked at it, the more I liked it.

Nina smiled, satisfied. "My boyfriend's coming today, but they won't let me redraw my eyebrows and they're all fucked up."

"Why do you gotta *draw* on your eyebrows?" Patty said.

"This bitch who was doing my eyebrows fucked them up!" Nina shot. "She fucked up one, and instead of telling me she just fucked up the other one too. And now they won't grow back so..." she motioned toward her forehead.

"They don't look that bad," Billie said. "And if he loves you, he won't care."

"Still, I don't want him to see me looking like this."

I tuned out the small talk to start painting over the crayon on my drawing. Washes of purple and brown on the tree trunk. Three different kinds of green for the fronds. A swish of red for the ground, so my subjects were not floating in an alien background of depthless white like me...

"NO, I CAN'T TAKE THAT! I CAN'T TAKE THAT!!!"

Shouting from the other end of the ward stopped all our drawing and beading cold, and Fiona stepped out to investigate.

It was the same voice that had startled me awake a few hours ago.

"Fuck, it's that pregnant chick again," sighed Nina.

"What?" I said, alarmed.

The yelling continued. "IT'LL HURT THE BABY!"

"She's not actually pregnant," Billie explained.

"She's just fat," Patty added, laughing a little.

"But she thinks she's pregnant," Billie said, "because they took her babies away. And that really messes with your head. So I guess this is how she's dealing with it."

"That's awful," I said. "And no one's talking to her?"

"Talk to her?" Nina scoffed. "Nah, here they just drug you up until you're quiet, like Brenda here. And Delilah." She shoved her thumb in Delilah's direction. She had been staring off into space, completely unaware of her name being mentioned.

"Yeah, you can't let them see you cry either, or else they'll never let you out," Billie explained. "If you want to cry, you have to do it in your shower."

"Seriously?" What they were saying made my throat feel immediately tight. No one said more, which meant, *yes, seriously.*

Down the hall, the yells slowly tapered out.

"There," Nina said. "They probably gave her a booty shot!"

"*A booty shot?*" crowed Angelique.

"Yeah, you know, the shot they give 'em to chill out!"

"I know," Angelique giggled, "but you can't call it a booty shot!"

"What," Nina defended, laughing along with the rest of us. "That's what it is!"

"Booty shots for all of us!" Patty laughed.

Billie grinned. "Yeah, for all the crazy kooks! Look!" And from a pile of stuff on the table, she pulled out a pair of the mesh underwear and pulled them onto her head. "Look at me, I'm *crazy!*"

"Let me try," Angelique said, pulling them onto her own head and then giving us a little pout.

"Oh, give it to Patty," Nina urged. "Bet it'll look cute on her."

And it did—she looked like a little elf with her yellow hair poking out from underneath and the edges of the underwear making corners like a distorted chef's hat.

"Don't let Gertrude see us or she'll think we're making fun of her!"

"Why?" I asked. "Who's that?"

"She's the Black lady that paces all day," Billie said.

"She was wearing underwear on her head yesterday—we don't know why," Nina explained, then lowered her voice. "We're not really sure what her deal is."

"God, I'd really go psycho in here if it weren't for all of you," Billie said solemnly. "I'm glad you're all here. I mean, I'm *not*—it's just—it was awful before we all hung out. And there were no groups and we all just stayed in our rooms."

"How long have you been here?" I asked her.

"Twelve days. Twelve *fucking days* in this shithole."

"Fuck."

"They keep giving me extra days 'cause I give 'em hell. I advocate for everyone else and cause trouble, so they keep punishing me."

"It's true," Nina said. "They're toughest on Billie. I give 'em a little trouble, but I don't ever get anything for it."

"Honey, that's 'cause you're young!" Billie said loudly,

gesticulating widely. "And cute! I'm old and loud."

"I'm thirty-nine," Nina said defensively, "and I was on dope for fifteen years so I know I'm not that cute. But I used to be. I used to have a real nice body. Aaaand then I had four kids." People laughed and then she turned to me. "How old are you, honey?"

"I'm twenty-three."

"Oh, damn, I thought you were younger."

"I'm nineteen," Angelique added and Nina pretended to spit out her coffee.

"You're a baby!"

"Whateverrr!"

Billie noticed my nearly-completed painting and started fawning over it, calling me an artistic genius. I shrugged, more out of uncaring than modesty, and offered to make her something to liven up her room.

"If you put it in the window, the sun should light it up pretty nicely," I said.

Billie blew me a kiss and I smiled.

I never thought keeping my sanity would come down to Crayola crayons. More quickly than I would have believed, time in the ward started to feel endless. I filled as many of the hours as I could stand by sketching in dozens of coloring book pages. But despite what the surge of adult coloring book sales would suggest, I did not find it very therapeutic.

After our allotted time with the art supplies was up, the social skills group began. Fiona rolled her cart away and was replaced by a bearded man in his late-twenties who introduced himself as Sayed. In his weak, tinny voice, he asked us our names and wrote them down on a piece of paper.

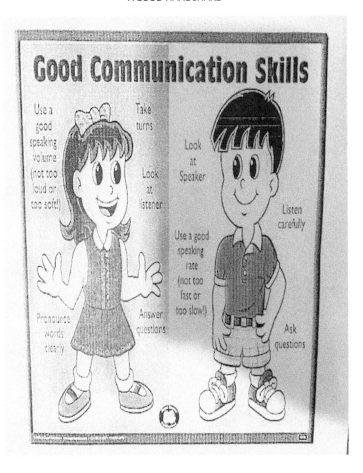

"We'll be talking about our communication skills today," Sayed announced, distributing worksheets to each of us. As the pages each fluttered down in front of us, we marveled at the content, aghast.

Is he joking?

On one side, two bug-eyed cartoon children, each with four fingers and oversized smiles, were pictured underneath the

39

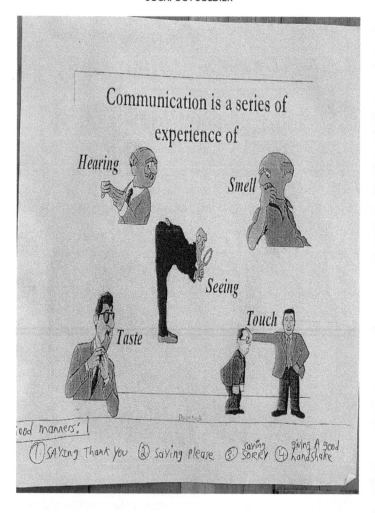

title, "Good Communication Skills." Phrases like *take turns* and *pronounce words clearly* surrounded them. On the other side, mismatched clipart people demonstrated the five senses below the words "Communication is a series of experience of." My inner editor raged.

The very bottom of the page was the best part though.

Before photocopying, someone had written in barely legible handwriting, "Good manners: (1) saying thank you (2) saying please (3) saying sorry (4) giving a good handshake."

Angelique voiced my inner thoughts. "This was written for, like, Kindergarteners," she seethed.

In a louder voice, Billie echoed her sentiment, saying, "Are you fucking serious, Sayed? Do you think we're stupid?"

He raised his hands defensively. "Let's just give it a chance, okay?"

Just then, Mia wandered in, bleary-eyed, and took a seat next to me. We handed her a worksheet, and she raised her eyebrows until they were almost touching her short bangs.

Thank God she came.

"Okay, everyone," Sayed said, trying to get the room's attention. "Can I get a volunteer to read the advice around good communication skills?"

And each of the juvenile phrases was recited aloud, in various tones of disbelief. I did not make eye contact with anyone, worried that I would burst out laughing, especially when Billie read with forced enthusiasm, "Use a good speaking rate! Not too fast or too slow!"

"Great, ladies," Sayed said. "Does anyone have any comments to make?"

Mia raised her hand but did not wait to be called on. "Can I just 'communicate' that I think these are some *very* good points. Especially since while we're in here, it's just *so* important for us to *communicate*."

Sayed, oblivious to her sarcasm, coaxed her on. "Thank you, Mia. Do you mind taking us through the other side?"

"*Sure*," Mia simpered. "Well, as everyone can see, it's very important that we use our sense of *smell* when we communi-

41

cate. Like earlier, we could *smell* that someone really didn't want to be here."

Some people snorted. Confused, I turned to Patty, who informed me that earlier, someone had been farting up a storm in the dayroom. It had caused something of an evacuation.

"And," Mia continued, "we could *smell* that some people aren't showering very often."

Others started to catch on to Mia's drift and looked back down at their worksheet for inspiration.

"And we can certainly *hear* when people communicate that they don't want to be here," Billie said.

"Yeah," Mia added. "And the breakfast this morning *tasted* like the chefs wanted to communicate—"

Sayed interrupted nervously. "What about some examples of *positive* communication?" he asked, his tone clearly trying to stay upbeat and undeterred.

"Sorry, Sayed," Nina said. "I just don't see much positive communication happening on this worksheet. I mean, the 'touch' guy is like gouging out the eyeball of that other guy!"

"Yeah!" Patty agreed. "And the 'taste' guy' is—is he eating his tie?"

Everyone was sniggering now and making snide comments to their neighbors. Facetious comments flew from every direction of the room, and even people like Francine and Delilah were enjoying us ham it up. I could not keep my eyes off Sayed, who was valiantly trying to keep us focused on the subject. It made me think he had chosen this worksheet himself, and therefore legitimately thought he might have produced a fruitful counseling session from it.

Mia was the best at keeping her face straight. "Guys," she said, expression deadpan, "let's really try and listen to what

Sayed is telling us."

A half-dozen incredulous faces turned to her.

"After all," Mia sang, "good manners are all about—" and her eyes scanned to the bottom of the worksheet to read, "—*saying thank you* and *giving a good handshake*."

"That's right, that's right," Sayed said, but Mia was not done.

"So let's all tell Sayed 'thank you' for teaching us about good communication."

And following her lead, we extended our hands in mock-handshake form and recited in sing-songy voices, "*Thank you, Sayed!*"

Finally understanding that he would never have our full attention or respect during this session, Sayed backed out of the room slowly while we cackled and high-fived. Mia leaned back in her seat triumphantly, crinkling up her worksheet and tossing it into the trash where it belonged.

6

Under Observation Does Not Mean Observed

Even before coming here, I had imagined what it would be like to be under psychiatric observation. Pop culture had given me a good amount of material to draw from. *Girl, Interrupted* suggested it would be easy to break out. *Legion* proposed that our uniforms might indicate our threat level. Most examples painted some picture of barely-contained tranquility.

So I figured a psych ward would be clean and white, with many therapists to talk to the quiet, medicated people brooding in their rooms.

Well, I was right about the medicated part.

Damn, were we medicated.

But this place was far from clean. I do not think I have ever felt grimier in my life. The floors were layered in gray dust and all the table surfaces were slightly tacky. Poor old Carla, with her OCD—I do not know how she withstood it.

And it certainly was not quiet. Someone was always yelling or talking back loudly to a counselor or banging on a wall. Even during quiet hours, every day from 3:00 to 4:00 p.m., noise and frenzy filled the ward. Quiet hours were a joke and just meant that we were required to "rest" in our individual rooms. But they were at least consistent; the nurses and counselors strictly enforced them in order to get a break from us. I imagine it is the same reason preschool teachers love naptime.

When I was back in my room after the two activities meant to be group therapy, I tasked myself with finding a way to stick my giraffe to the window. The page would not lean on the glass on its own since the vent was blowing air right below it. I tried using toothpaste as glue, but it was not gummy enough. The Vaseline I had been given worked well enough, and I used two dabs in the corner to stick it in place.

I stood back and admired my handiwork, but the two seconds of pride were deflated by the thought that this meant—*shit!*—I was settling in. Though maybe my artwork was not even permanent. Billie had warned me that the counselors might call it a fire hazard and take it down.

"But that doesn't stop them from letting us put up pictures in the dayroom," she had said. "Go figure."

One of the orderlies came by with a cart full of pills and water cups and said my blood test results had indicated low potassium levels. He said I had to drink this electric orange beverage, about a shot's worth, in order to get them up.

"Some people say it tastes bad so I'm going to mix it with this orange juice, okay?" He stirred the two liquids together and handed me the cup.

All I knew about potassium was that it's in bananas, so I guess I figured the potassium stuff would taste like that. I took a huge gulp and nearly spat it out. Apart from not liking orange juice in the first place, the potassium shit tasted like heavily saturated saltwater.

"I need some water," I gasped to the orderly.

"When you finish it."

I shook my head. "Nuh-uh. Now. I need to take it in turns."

He sighed like this was some huge burden and poured water into a tiny Styrofoam cup from a bigger Styrofoam cup. "Come on," he urged.

"I could have just taken it without the juice," I retorted, then took another sip as big as I could stand without gagging.

God, it tasted horrible—salt and citrus. And the texture had changed too, into something more viscous and almost gooey. Awful!

About five swigs in, my nose started bleeding again. Unlike earlier, I did not catch it in time. I managed to safeguard the cup but got huge bloody splatters on my pants and the linoleum. The orderly, suddenly energized, ran for something to mop up the mess, so I just stood there with my face toward the ceiling tiles, feeling the blood slowly ooze down the left side of my face.

Blood tastes better than salty orange juice, in case you were wondering.

"Here," the orderly said when he returned, thrusting a few Kleenexes (where did he get those?) at me. I got out of his way as he wiped up the drops on the floor.

"Sorry," I apologized, the tissue wedged into my nostril. "I don't know why my nose has been bleeding."

He did not acknowledge it—just threw the stained tissues into my paper bag trash bins. "Did you finish drinking?"

"Oh, yeah." I had one big gulp left and I tipped it into the side of my mouth so the Kleenex wouldn't soak it up. "Done."

The orderly pushed his cart down the hall, and I went to my bathroom to snort out the blood clot. As I was leaning over the sink, I thought about how the guy had not asked a single medical question about the fact I had now had two nose bleeds before noon. I know bloody noses are not exactly life-threatening, but still.

As I finished cleaning myself up, a tall and pretty young woman in a yellow cardigan tapped on my door.

"Hi, you busy?" she said in a clear-as-a-bell voice. "Can I talk to you for a sec?"

I held out my arm towards my open room.

"I'm Caroline, your social worker," she said. She extended her hand and confirmed my full name. She could not have been much older than me, and I felt extra scrubby and self-conscious in my hospital pants and wrinkled tee shirt. Surely my hair was a mess. Hers was long and straight and sleek and *fuck.*

"Hi," I said, sniffing. My nose still felt pulpy.

Caroline's face was bright but she crumpled it into an empathetic expression. "So you got here last night, huh? How are things?"

"Fine. The other patients are nice."

"Good!"

I nodded.

"My job," Caroline explained, "is to make sure you're doing okay in here and that you have a good plan of action for when you get out. Do you currently see a psychiatrist?"

I told her no, that I had been getting my meds from my primary care physician since moving to Chicago.

"How about a therapist?"

Again, I told her no, but that I had seen one regularly in the past, including when I first moved to Chicago. I had stopped seeing that one when I started traveling Monday through

Thursday for work. Most therapists did not take patients on the weekends, and the idea of sacrificing Friday happy hours for therapy had never stuck.

"Yikes. Well, if it's okay with you, how about I look for therapists that are taking patients on weekends in your neighborhood? How's that sound? And I can make an appointment with a psychiatrist for you that your insurance covers. Sound good?"

"Sounds good."

And it did. It would save me an hour on Google and an afternoon of frustrating phone calls. I knew I had been lax on the mental healthcare front—it was just so easy to let that slip when work was busy and Life was happening.

I told her which neighborhood I lived in and then asked if someone had been able to get ahold of my friend or manager, both of whom were probably worried, or at least curious, by now. She informed me that yes, Mackenzie had been able to reach both of them. Then she smiled, shook my hand again, and left. It was not a long visit, but I felt better knowing she would handle future appointments for me. It helped that she acted like she was made of sunshine too. That shit rubs off on you.

An orderly came in to take my blood pressure again, and then I was back to sitting in my room, wondering what I was supposed to be doing. It occurred to me that no one had really given me a formal introduction to the ward to tell me what the schedule was, what we were supposed to be doing here to heal, or when I would be seeing a psychiatrist to talk about any sort of treatment plan. I figured someone like Mackenzie or Caroline would come by and give me some kind of orientation, but no one ever did.

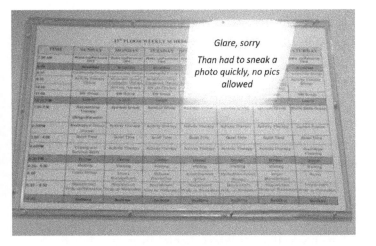

I wandered to the nearest posted schedule and tried to sync what I had done that morning with what was printed in fading ink. Arts and Crafts with Fiona must have been Community Group unless it was supposed to have been Activity Therapy and the time was just off. Then that abomination of a session with Sayed must have been an attempt at Expressive Therapy. The schedule said that right now at 11:30 a.m. we were supposed to be in the middle of "SW Group." I had to guess what the letters stood for—social work? Second wind? Super women? No one was in either dayroom, so I had nobody to ask and concluded that it must not be happening. So far, we were two for four on the schedule.

Out of sheer boredom, I took some laps around the floor. Another woman was doing laps in the opposite direction as me, and although I left her plenty of space, she always seemed to veer closer to my path but never made eye contact. Sometimes she hummed and once she careened into me and pushed me aside. If she had not been clearly disturbed or if it had not been my first day on the floor, I might have said something. Instead, I just started walking in the same direction as her and made sure we were always separated by a length of hallway.

I started peeking into rooms to look for Mia. I wanted to ask if anyone had given *her* an orientation spiel. When I finally found her, she was curled in her bed, clearly asleep. I made a note to ask her the next time I saw her—maybe someone had just forgotten to give it to me.

I paced and wandered for a while, but there was not much to explore. I went back to my bed and tossed and turned until I heard the lunchtime commotion.

Lunch was like breakfast. Same silver cart. Same table in Dayroom A. Same comment from Nina about it tasting like ass. My uncustomized tray of chicken enchiladas, overcooked green, beans and, once again, lukewarm decaf coffee went mostly untouched.

Mia finally made it out of her room and asked about who had been yelling earlier.

"Earlier today or earlier last night?" Billie said.

"Just ignore the yells," Nina advised. "It's usually nothing."

I leaned over toward Mia and asked if anyone had spoken with her yet.

"What do you mean?"

"Like, to tell you what's going on. How long we're here and stuff?"

"Nope."

"And don't expect them too," Billie said, hearing us. "They're not great at giving out information. But what do you need to know?"

I looked at her energized and helpful face and gaped, unsure what to ask. She filled in the silence for me.

50

"Most people aren't here too long," she said comfortingly. "But it depends. Ask your doctor when you see them. Hopefully you have a good one."

"There's really nobody that tells us this stuff?" I said. "That doesn't seem right."

"That's not the only thing," Patty said, poking her food with her fork.

"This food is disgusting," Mia declared.

I agreed. I poked my food around the tray a bit and then offered it to anyone who wanted it. Big Brenda took me up on my offer but was too dazed to actually get it into her mouth. I returned my tray and lumbered back to bed, wrapping the sheets around myself so that everything I saw was white.

I was *so bored*. I sat in my cocoon and tried not to think about Sad Things, but there were so many Sad Things I could think about. My mind was a menu of depressing thoughts, and in my boredom, each black hole seemed almost appetizing.

Just after 1:00 p.m., a distraction finally presented itself in the form of a voice yelling, "Grooooup!"

It was Spiritual Group, which people seemed generally excited about. Not many were in the dayroom—most were napping, I guessed—but Billie, Nina, Angelique, Patty, Francine, Little Brenda, and Carla were there. Personally, I am not religious, but I was not about to go back to pacing the halls with bumper-car-lady. Besides, the hospital socks had uncomfortable square toes, and walking in them just made me more aware of that fact.

The group was led by a well-intended chaplain with wire-rimmed glasses and, unlike with Fiona and Sayed earlier in the day, everyone was giving him their full attention.

"I don't consider myself that religious," Billie was saying

to the chaplain, "but I do appreciate you being here and I appreciate you talking to us like we're not animals."

"Well, the Lord asks that we treat each other with respect."

"Yeah, they're real respectful in here," scoffed Billie sarcastically. "Did you know, I saw Dr. Dizon the other day and you know what he did? You know what? He knocked my *Mi Shebeirach* right to the ground. I had it all written out, see, and he just knocked it right to the ground. He *laughed* and he said 'ha! We're not Jewish,' and pushed it off the table! And the nurse that was in there with him just laughed too—can you believe that?"

"I'm so sorry to hear that," the chaplain said, shaking his head.

"They treat us like *fuck-ing a-ni-mals*," Billie huffed. "No respect."

"Would it make you feel better if we read from the bible?" He held out a navy blue paper copy of the New Testament.

"I mean, I'm not religious," Billie said again. "But yeah, maybe it would."

Nina interjected, "Ooh! Can I recite somethin'?"

"Go ahead," the chaplain said generously, leaning back in his chair.

Nina lit up. "I know all sorts of verses. You guys want Matthew? Psalms? I know *'The Lord is my shepherd, I shall not be in want. He makes me lie down in green pastures, he leads me beside quiet waters, he restores my soul.'*"

"I know that one too," Angelique said.

Nina continued, "And I know Philippians 4:13, *'I can do all things through Christ who strengthens me,'* and *'Trust in the Lord with all your heart and lean not on your own understanding.'* Y'all, I could go on all day. Don't get me started on the Lord!"

"I know some poems," Francine said sweetly from her wheelchair and started to recite, "*I can do all things through Christ who strengthens me.*"

"I just said that, silly," Nina said.

"Does anyone want to read something?" the Chaplain offered to the table at large. "Or we can talk about faith and how it helps us heal?"

"Can I tell everyone how I met Christ?" Nina said. "Sorry, y'all. I don't mean to take over."

"I'd like to hear that," Billie said.

"Yeah, me too," Angelique agreed.

And with a smile on her face, Nina launched into a wonderful story about how she used to not know God until a religious friend of hers invited her to work at a church event. "And there was this woman there and she pulled me aside and told me that she knew. She knew I was struggling and that I needed help, and she knew all these things about me—all these things—and they were the exact same sorts of things I used to pray to God about only I didn't think he was listening. And that's when I knew he's real and that his love is real, 'cause how else would she have known all that stuff?"

"I've been a Christian forever," Little Brenda interposed, drawing a hurt look from Nina's face.

"It's true, we all find the Lord at different times," the chaplain said diplomatically. "The important thing is that we find him at some point in our lives and give ourselves to him."

"Some people worship false idols," Little Brenda argued.

Billie turned her body to Little Brenda and opened her mouth, but the Chaplain intervened with a well-timed, "Shall we pray?"

We clasped hands and prayed, and then Spiritual Group was over. Patty made eye contact with me during the prayer and started giggling, but Nina, Angelique, Francine, and even Carla all said 'Amen' at the end.

"Y'all done in here?" came a call from the door. It was one of the counselors, a curvy Black woman with dark pink lipstick and short twists, pushing Fiona's silver craft cart. In addition to the beads and coloring sheets, there was now a shiny bingo set too.

"Venetia!" Billie cried. "Are we playing bingo?"

"Yep. I don't know where y'all's other group counselor is, so I figured I'd run it if that's okay."

"Sure, that's okay!" Billie said, enthusiastically. "Here, I can help you set up—wait, let me see if some of the other girls want to play."

"Are there prizes?" Nina asked.

"Yeah," Venetia answered, nodding at a paper bag in the cart. "Got 'em in here. Snacks good?"

"Snacks *great*. I'm starved."

We all said goodbye and thank you to the chaplain and began dispersing bingo cards and plastic chips. Billie came back in with Big Brenda and Mia, while Carla slipped away. Mia sat next to me with four bingo cards in front of her, while most others grabbed two or three. I grabbed two—my mind was still feeling sluggish and I did not think I could keep track of four sets at once.

Venetia began to call out the bingo numbers, repeating each one twice. Most of us listened intently and placed our colored bingo chips eagerly. Francine just looked happy to be there with us, and Big Brenda continued to nod off. When Angelique had a spare second between calls of "B-10!" and "G-51!" she

54

would place Brenda's chips for her.

Billie was the first to win, but we kept playing on our boards, and so Mia and I came in second only a few more calls after. Our prize options were packets of Lorna Doone cookies, one hundred calorie packs of Oreo crisps, and bags of white cheddar popcorn. I opted for the cookies and cleared my board, thinking how great these would taste with lukewarm decaf coffee.

The rhythm of Venetia's calls, sometimes punctuated with cries of "Bingo!" " filled the dayroom. A couple other women wandered in and perused through the coloring pages.

Soon, I won another round, and when we did not clear our boards after, I got a third bingo with the very next call. But the snacks were running low, so I only took one more pack of Lorna Doone's, even though Nina insisted I had earned two more.

"Two's enough for me," I assured her.

I tired of bingo pretty quickly. While the rest of the gals geared up for rounds five, six, seven and eight, I spied a newspaper at the other end of the room. It had been heavily rifled through and was two days old, but thankfully, no one had nabbed the crossword.

In Real Life, I did the LA Times crossword every day, partly out of compulsive habit and partly because I heard once that it helps ward off dementia and who wants that. It was a treat to find a crossword here, and since it was a Wednesday crossword, I figured I could at least fill most of it in.

I took it back to my room and then realized I did not have a pen.

Popping my head out of the door, I asked the counselor on guard, Yulia, if she had a pen or pencil that I could use. Yulia was a thin woman with harshly dyed blonde hair and wide brown eyes. She looked at me like I was nuts, and I realized why. Right—pens were sharp objects. Potential weapons.

"I can give you a crayon," she offered.

You cannot do a crossword with a fucking crayon. I smiled tightly and replied, "Sure."

She opened the locked closet behind her and then handed me the blue. "It's the sharpest one," she said apologetically.

"Thanks. It'll probably work."

I thought about how much it must suck to work in a place like this, where all the patients viewed you as either a nuisance or an enemy. Based on what I had already seen and heard, some counselors were definitely assholes. Then others, like Yulia, genuinely seemed nice. Or at least, like they wanted to be nice. But working here day in and day out must really grind a person down.

One of the clues from that day's puzzle was a five-letter word for "drench." I filled in D-R-O-W-N as neatly as I could with the crayon. The night before had indeed felt like drowning, and that first day still felt a bit like that, but for a different reason. Instead of all my anxieties being focused on the past or future, they were now fixated on the very, very present.

The yelling, the terrible food, the general griminess—I understood some of those things had to come part and parcel with being in an under-resourced psychiatric institution. But the explicit lack of legitimate therapy and quality medical care had to be approaching malpractice.

It was just after 2:00 p.m. on my first day and I was starting to realize that this was it. Health professionals would come for mere moments and counseling would be delivered by glorified babysitters.

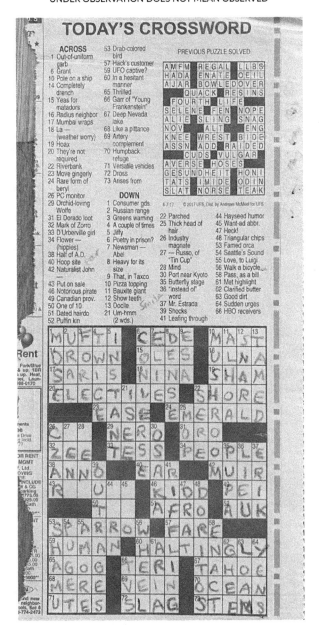

TODAY'S CROSSWORD

ACROSS
1 Out-of-uniform garb
6 Grant
10 Pole on a ship
14 Completely drench
15 Yeas for matadors
16 Radius neighbor
17 Mumbai wraps
18 La — (weather worry)
19 Hoax
20 They're not required
22 Riverbank
23 Move gingerly
24 Rare form of beryl
26 PC monitor
29 Orchid-loving Wolfe
31 El Dorado loot
32 Mark of Zorro
33 D'Urberville girl
34 Flower — (hippies)
38 Half of A.D.
40 Hoop site
42 Naturalist John
43 Put on sale
46 Notorious pirate
49 Canadian prov.
50 One of 10
51 Dated hairdo
52 Puffin kin

53 Drab-colored bird
57 Hack's customer
59 UFO captive?
60 In a hesitant manner
65 Thrilled
66 Garr of "Young Frankenstein"
67 Deep Nevada lake
68 Like a pittance
69 Artery complement
70 Humpback refuge
71 Versatile vehicles
72 Dross
73 Arises from

DOWN
1 Consumer gds.
2 Russian range
3 Greens warning
4 A couple of times
5 Jiffy
6 Poetry in prison?
7 Newsman — Abel
8 Heavy for its size
9 That, in Taxco
10 Pizza topping
11 Bauxite giant
12 Show teeth
13 Docile
21 Um-hmm (2 wds.)

22 Parched
25 Thick head of hair
26 Industry magnate
27 — Russo, of "Tin Cup"
28 Mind
30 Port near Kyoto
35 Butterfly stage
36 "Instead of" word
37 Mr. Estrada
39 Shocks
41 Leafing through

44 Hayseed humor
45 Want-ad abbr.
47 Heck!
48 Triangular chips
53 Famed orca
54 Seattle's Sound
55 Love, to Luigi
56 Walk a bicycle, e.g.
58 Pass, as a bill
61 Met highlight
62 Clarified butter
63 Good dirt
64 Sudden urges
66 HBO receivers

PREVIOUS PUZZLE SOLVED

A	M	F	M		R	E	G	A	L		L	L	B	S
H	A	D	A		E	N	A	T	E		O	E	I	L
A	J	A	R		B	O	W	L	E	D	O	V	E	R
		Q	U	A	C	K		R	E	S	I	N	S	
F	O	U	R	T	H		L	I	F	E				
S	E	L	E	N	E		F	E	N		N	O	P	E
A	L	I	E		S	L	I	N	G		S	N	A	G
N	O	V		A	L	T		E	N	G				
K	N	E	E		W	R	E	S	T		B	I	D	E
A	S	S	N		A	D	D		R	A	I	D	E	D
				C	U	D	S		V	U	L	G	A	R
A	V	E	R	S	E		H	O	S	E	S			
G	E	S	U	N	D	H	E	I	T		H	O	N	I
T	A	T	S		I	M	I	D	E		O	D	I	N
S	L	A	T		N	O	R	S	E		T	E	A	K

6-7-17   © 2017 UFS, Dist. by Andrews McMeel for UFS

M	U	F	T	I		C	E	D	E		M	A	S	T
D	R	O	W	N		O	L	E	S		U	L	N	A
S	A	R	I	S		N	I	N	A		S	H	A	M
E	L	E	C	T	I	V	E	S		S	H	O	R	E
		E	A	S	E		E	M	E	R	A	L	D	
C	C			N	E	R	O		O	R	O			
Z	E	E		T	E	S	S		P	E	O	P	L	E
A	N	N	O		E	A	R		M	U	I	R		
R	U		U			K	I	D	D		P	E	I	
	T				A	F	R	O		A	U	K		
S	P	A	R	R	O	W		F	A	R	E			
H	U	M	A	N		H	A	L	T	I	N	G	L	Y
A	G	O	G		E	R	I		T	A	H	O	E	
M	E	R	E		V	E	I	N		O	C	E	A	N
U	T	E	S		S	L	A	G		S	T	E	M	S

57

Would I ever know what was really going on?

And in here, how the hell was I supposed to get Capital-B Better?

Maybe that was not the point. Maybe this place was just another battle to overcome, another trauma to endure. Maybe instead of focusing on satisfaction, I should instead focus on survival. If I had just landed myself in a war zone, I would take up arms.

Eight-letter word for "poetry in prison"? C-O-N-V-E-R-S-E.

Five-letter word for "UFO captive"? H-U-M-A-N.

Four-letter word for "Heck!"? D-R-A-T.

7

Poetry

I had my first notable mental health breakdown in my junior year of high school. My intention had been to commit suicide on a Sunday night, Easter, but then I delayed. I wanted to see my friends and teachers one last time. The morning before I left for school on Monday, I wrote The Note, set up The Pills, and braced myself for The Last Day.

But a funny thing happened in the middle of the school day—regret. Paralyzing regret. I had not even done anything yet, but knowing that the stage was set up made me feel like once I went home, I would have no choice but to carry it through. I did not want to kill myself—I just wanted the pain to stop.

I was in Ms. Cardona's Poetry class when everyone filed out for the lunch dismissal. The crowd bustled away toward the lunchroom, and I floated behind them, eyes blank, feet shuffling. I only made it a few steps beyond the door before crumpling in the empty hallway. And since my classmates were either all in the cafeteria or still in classrooms, no one saw me in crisis.

I knew a group of friends was hanging out in Mr. Motes's empty room a few doorways down. With all the strength I could muster, I crawled on my hands and knees, shaking, tears streaming down my face, and kicked at the door until someone came to investigate.

I could not talk that time either—I had been too afraid I would scream or start sobbing openly—so one of the guys grabbed a pen and paper. He and I had been friends since Kindergarten and had grown significantly apart in the later years of school, but as I scribbled down the scary one-word thoughts floating in my head, he put his hand on my shoulder and tried to understand.

From my tears and the few legible words like 'Pills' and 'Help,' the guys solved the puzzle. And until an adult arrived, four of them sat with me on the carpet, as I wept, devastated but not alone, against the doorframe of Mr. Motes's classroom.

That was the first time I Got Help. 'Help' meant that I was ushered to the school counselor's office, where Home was called, and my boyfriend at the time was contacted so he could sit with me until my dad arrived. The next day I had a crisis psychiatric appointment where it was decided I was stable enough for an outpatient program, meaning I could still go to Prom in a few weeks. I slept and watched movies and made collages out of magazines before returning to school a few days later. No one was any the wiser—they just thought I caught a spring flu.

One of the collages I had made during my "vacation" was really just a poem fashioned out of colorful words cut from magazines. I had pasted it onto a piece of giant yellow poster board and brought the finished work to my poetry class. Ms. Cardona hung it up in the back of the classroom for the rest of the school year, until I asked for it back so I could tack it to my bedroom ceiling.

Ms. Cardona was one of those life-changing teachers that students take to, especially those with artistic souls looking for solace in language and poetry. I took two classes with her: AP Language & Composition and then a poetry class a year later. I was also lucky enough to have her as a homeroom teacher, which meant every two weeks I got to sit at the front of her classroom and pretend to listen to whatever administrative announcement she was obligated to share. But I respected the hell out of her. She was genuine in all her interactions and gave it to us straight. Her feedback on our writing was constructive and never more than we could handle. She gave creative assignments, like the time she asked us to create and contribute to a blog for the semester. And she had a nostril piercing.

After I returned to school from my "vacation," her poetry class became part of my counseling. She shepherded us to the most resonant poems and passages, and I was able to use other people's elegiac words to better understand pain, beauty, love, and life. At the end of the school year, we put the desks in a circle and read out loud our favorite poems. I looked at each of the seniors in that class, all a year ahead of me on the brink of graduation, and shared my poem about being brave and not fearing failure even when an unsettled mind does its best to convince you of all the ways you could fail.

When I gave my class's graduation speech a year later, Ms. Cardona was the one I asked to introduce me on stage. She started her introduction by quoting the poem I had written the year earlier. It set my soul alight.

Ms. Cardona taught me that poetry and art make life

beautiful—no matter how painful and ugly life gets, there is still beauty to be found. It can be found in friendship, in sunshine, in serendipity—sometimes you have to look hard, but there is always something, somewhere.

Looking around my psych ward room, I was struggling to find any sort of beauty in the drab beige-ness. Even the goofy, cartoonish giraffe I had painted, though colorful, did little to bring light into the room. So I closed my eyes and tried to imagine beautiful things instead. The sparkle of late afternoon light on Lake Michigan. Murals and street art. Families eating ice cream together. Rainbows.

It was quiet hours and there was nothing better to do than drift into a restless, uncomfortable sleep. When I woke up sweaty and dazed, I could feel another stream of blood deep in my nasal passage. I would get bloody noses fairly often, but never three times in a day. It was *that* dry in the ward.

I pinched the bridge of my nose and waited until it felt safe, then took another go at the crossword with my now-dull blue crayon. Since the bed was not against the wall, I had nothing to lean against, so I sat on the floor, propped the pillow between myself and the textured wallpaper, and used the ground as a hard surface under the newspaper.

I tried to ignore the scattering of yells from the opposite end of the ward. Hearing those screams made my skin crawl—I wanted to cover up my ears and drown out the sound with my own shrieks of torment. Were the demons they were fighting imaginary or real?

Remembering that phone hours started at 5:00 p.m., I traipsed into the hall to check the time. The clock above the counselor on guard's head reported 4:50 p.m., meaning I had slept for almost two hours.

At least that was one way to pass the time.

Already it felt like I had been here for days, but it had only been seventeen hours—not even a full day! Yesterday at this time, I had been replying to emails in the comfort of my own apartment, with access to hot coffee, fresh air, and a purring cat.

Since I had no official information on what my stay would be like or when I could be discharged, I felt vastly uninformed and anxiety bubbled within me. Just like during my days in school, I wanted to get my hands on the syllabus—to know what would be on the test so I could figure out how to pass it with flying colors. Who was I supposed to be trying to impress? Who did I need to convince that I was functional and "fixed"?

High-functioning depression is a tricky beast to spot in the wild. Unless I told you plainly, you might never know I was severely depressed. I was always in the top of my class, competitive to a fault and fiercely independent. I tackled heavy workloads and excelled under pressure. I traveled often and went out with friends. I am not sure what most people's mental image of a depressed person is—maybe sweatpants?—but I would understand if I did not fit it with my dimpled smile, colorful dresses, and typical air of confidence.

But there are still signs. Even for people with high-functioning depression, there are always, always signs. Medical websites list signs like these:

- Difficulty sleeping
- Sleeping more than usual
- Changes in appetite
- Withdrawal from social interaction
- Loss of interest in things that used to be pleasurable

- Lack of energy
- Feelings of worthlessness
- Difficulty concentrating or remembering things

Those are all good and true—but many of those are hard to spot in a loved one because they are so internal, or because they manifest behind closed doors or outside social hours. Here are the behaviors I wish people were aware of because they are indicative of some of the signs above:

- Canceling on plans, especially more than usual
- Spending more time in my room than normal
- Stopping in the middle of what I am doing as if I have lost my train of thought
- Talking slower than normal or less than normal
- Frequently mentioning how tired I am—or looking extremely tired

My friends could spot many of those signs, and once they did, they greeted me with their time and company. As I stared at the walls of my beige room, I realized that those friendships were the thing of beauty I could fixate on. There is always beauty to be found, and I knew at that moment I needed to find my friends. Or rather, since I was locked in a psych ward, they needed to find me.

8

Soup & The Soul

"So I'm in the psych ward."

No immediate response from Than on the other side of the line.

"And I'm *fine*," I assured him. "But yeah, I'm here."

I had finally gotten ahold of him after, promptly at 5:00 p.m., I asked the blonde-bobbed counselor on guard if I could use the phone. I thought it would be a stationary wall unit and imagined a rotary dial. Instead, I was handed a thick gray cell phone, like an old Nokia but some other make, with a rubber band around the middle to keep the back panel in.

"Dial 9 first," Beth had told me.

So I dialed 9 and then the digits to Than's phone, which is one of the few numbers I have memorized. I hit the green phone button, but nothing happened. I tried twice more.

"Excuse me," I said to Beth, feeling dumb. "It's not working for me."

"What's the area code?"

And I had told her.

"You can only dial '312,' '872,' and '773' codes from that."

"Um, okay. So what should I do?"

"Dial 0."

"So call the operator?" I clarified, getting exasperated but trying to stay even.

"Yeah, that's what I just said."

The first time the operator patched me through, I had gotten Than's voicemail. Knowing he had probably just ignored the number because it was unfamiliar, I dialed again and finally got him on the first ring. He was, as I had figured, slightly panicked.

"Jesus," he finally began. "Yeah, I left you a voicemail earlier 'cause I wasn't sure you came home last night."

Hearing his voice, I felt immediately guilty for any stress I had caused him. "Sorry—I don't have access to my phone. But someone said they got ahold of you this morning."

"Nope," he said. "Maybe they left a voicemail, but I wouldn't have checked it."

"Yeah, who checks voicemail?" I agreed, irked at Mackenzie if this was what she considered "successfully contacted." "Well, I'm okay," I repeated. "Visiting hours are from 6:30 to 8:00 p.m. I haven't seen a doctor yet, but who knows."

"I can visit tonight?"

"Yeah," I said. "I'll be here."

He paused, waiting, then said, "Um, where is there?"

And I realized that I had spent almost twenty-four hours not knowing where I was beside some hospital, somewhere in Chicago, on the fifteenth floor. "Oh right," I said, laughing a little and turning to Beth. "Where am I?"

She gave me a small smile, perhaps sympathetically but also possibly appreciating the humor in the situation. It was a crazy question to ask—only a true psychotic person or perhaps a coma patient should have the need to voice that query—but being treated like you are crazy will make you crazy. She told me the name of the hospital and the intersection; I relayed it to Than, who promised he would be there at 6:30 p.m.

"And can you bring me some clothes? And books? And cards, and my penguin?"

"Yeah, what clothes?"

"Soft stuff. Nothing with strings. Tee shirts, underwear, yoga pants." I told him which shelves and drawers he could find everything on and cringed internally at the thought of him going through my underwear drawer. But then I realized the alternative meant wearing my current pair or else mesh underwear for who knows how long. I pictured this morning, with Patty wearing that underwear on her head and smiled to myself.

We went back and forth on which books he would bring and then, as I saw other women eyeing the phone, I told him about the ten-minute limit. "See you later, then," he said.

"Yeah, bye."

Hanging up, I felt quite alone, which made no sense because now I had a definite visitor to look forward to. It was that sensation that comes so frequently with depression—feeling quite alone while surrounded by a sea of people. I was feeling it even in this loud and personality-filled psychiatric ward. I bet most of the other patients were probably feeling some version of this too.

It happens all the time when you least expect it. The debilitating loneliness, despite having friends, coworkers, family who *care*. And knowing they care—it still does not always do enough to breach the figurative gap that isolates you. Loneliness is an illusion—but a strong one.

I could talk my mind into a pit all day long and convince my-self that my friends could do without me, that my coworkers would forget about me, or that my family would get over the loss of me soon enough. But I know, *really*, that none of that is true. It's a battle, day in and day out, between loneliness and love, interrupted by the banality of things like—

"Dinner, ladies!"

The silver cart rolled toward me, where I was still sitting on the floor after taking my call and handing the phone to the next person. Taking a deep breath, I pushed my body up and got in the clump to await my tray.

A chicken breast, caked in now-damp spices. A cafeteria cup of orange sherbet. A carton of milk. A white scoop of mashed potatoes. A shallow bowl of what I was told was potato soup. And of course, decaf coffee and no plastic knife.

"How are we supposed to eat this without cutting it?" Billie was saying once we were all back at our table.

"Maybe they want us to choke," Mia joked.

"Brenda didn't even get silverware again!" Billie noticed. "It's a conspiracy against Brenda's, I swear! The other day, *this* Brenda—" and she pointed her finger to the elderly lady sitting at a different table, "—didn't get silverware either."

Someone else offered theirs up. "She can have mine. I'm not eating this shit."

"My sherbet's already melted," I marveled. "Anyone want it anyway?"

"Honey," Nina was saying to Delilah, "you gotta eat some-thin'. You haven't eaten all day."

"She could probably have the soup," Angelique suggested.

And so we placed a plastic spoon in Delilah's giant hand and watched, fascinated, as she started shoveling room temperature soup into her mouth at an astonishing pace.

The potatoes—sorry, I need to specify, the *mashed* potatoes—were nasty. I discovered if I dipped the mashed potatoes
in the potato soup-like gravy, both were semi-edible. The
chicken, even though it was a startling orange color from
whatever spices the kitchen had used, still managed to be
tasteless, and so I tried dipping that in the soup too.

I could not eat more than a few bites. At least the depressing
atmosphere had subdued my appetite.

Others at the table were eating more heartily. In fact, Billie
was eating with absolute gusto.

"What a great day," she said exuberantly. She told us that
she had just spoken with her ex-husband, a lawyer, who
thought he had found a way to get her out of there. "And
we had *four* groups today. Art, Spiritual, Bingo, and whatever
fucking Sayed's was supposed to be. *Four.*"

"Is that not typical?" I asked.

"Oh no. We usually have, like, *one.* Maybe two, if we're
lucky."

I raised my eyebrows, unimpressed. Wasn't the whole
purpose of a place like this to have therapy all day long? Even
criminally mediocre therapy, like Fiona's "art therapy," was
healthier than sitting in our rooms all day.

Suddenly Mia and Angelique both screamed. Creamy white
vomit was gurgling out of Delilah's mouth, and everyone
backed away from the table; a couple people ran straight out
of the room. I looked around for a counselor or a nurse, but
there was, unbelievably, no one besides us.

"Help!!!" Billie bellowed, running out toward the nurse's
station.

"Fuck, that's disgusting," Nina commented, throwing her

napkin in Delilah's direction.

But Delilah made no effort to stop the gushing spew that was still erupting out of her mouth. It puddled in her gown and splattered on the floor as the rest of us looked at each other, unsure of what to do.

"She didn't even chew it," Patty marveled.

Indeed, soupy potato chunks were swimming in the growing pool around Delilah's chair.

A staff member eventually came in, urged along by Billie, with Mia and Angelique tiptoeing in their wake. Trying not to gag, we helped clean up the spill, and the nurse ushered the still-silent Delilah back to her room.

"I can't even look at barf without..." Mia made a gagging motion and sat back down, far away from the damage. "And I'm definitely not eating *that*." She pushed her soup away and drew her knees up to her chest.

"Shit," Nina said, shaking her head. "I mean, what do they have her on? It must have really fucked her up if she can't even eat."

"You doing okay?" I asked Big Brenda, who had not moved during the whole ordeal.

"I'm good," she responded monotonously.

At least Big Brenda was still eating without much of a problem.

"That was SO! GROSS!" Angelique exclaimed.

"Disgusting," Billie affirmed. "And they didn't hurry to get in here when I told them!"

"Ew, I think I got some on my leg," Patty wailed.

"My God," Billie wondered, looking around at us. "What are we even doing here?"

From the other end of the room, the other Brenda, Old

Brenda, softly said, "I like it better here than the senior home."

That shut us all up.

"Yeah," Big Brenda said. "It's quieter here than at home."

Mia looked at me and raised her eyebrows, thinking the same thing I was: quieter *here*?

After an awkward silence, Nina finally broke the ice. "Yeah, I guess at least here we get to color all the fuckin' butterflies we want!"

"And the soup tastes *great*," I drawled sarcastically.

"Is anyone else still hungry?" Billie asked, but everyone shook their heads. One behind the other, we picked up our trays and returned them to the silver cart.

Than, true to his word, came punctually at 6:30 p.m. The staff had cleared out Dayroom B for visiting hours, which, un-like Dayroom A, had no patient-made artwork posted around the drab walls save for a picture of a toilet ripped out of a magazine on which someone had written in all caps, "YOU ARE NOT SHIT." The chairs were the same though, made of brown plastic and weighed down with sand so that we could not throw them in any potential fit of madness.

I told him a bit about my day, leaving out anything I thought might scare him but emphasizing that I had not seen a psy-chiatrist yet and had only seen a nurse practitioner for a few minutes with no warning. I told him that a lot of folks were nice and a lot of folks were also scary, but Than and I agreed that this was not surprising. We also agreed that referring to this place as 'the loony bin' was more fun than 'psychiatric ward' or, worse, 'adult behavioral center'.

Than let me know that a few of my friends from work had messaged him, asking where I was. Not being in the office on Friday meant that I had missed plans with them, which was unlike me, but I was touched to hear they had gone sleuthing on Facebook to get ahold of Than in order to ask about me. I let him know that he could tell them where I was, and they were welcome to visit if they were willing. Then we worked on my crayon-crossword together, like we used to do during college classes (except with *pens*). For a little bit, everything was normal. I forgot that I was not wearing a bra and that my socks were square and that I had slept the hours of a fussy baby. But too soon, staff members were ushering all the visitors out at 8:00 p.m. sharp.

As Than signed out in their pink binder, I was handed the items he had brought me, which had been inspected for sharp edges and contraband (and placed in yet another brown paper bag). I saw the clothes, the deck of cards, the books...

Noticing what was missing, I turned to Than. "My penguin?" This was the stuffed animal I had grown up with and, even as an adult, stayed on my bed. I had been hoping to use it as something to cuddle, or at least, as a second pillow option.

The counselor clucked, "You can't have it, miss."

"Why not? It's a stuffed animal."

And from another bag beside the binder, the counselor pointed to the grey knit scarf around my penguin's neck. "It's not allowed."

I was too incredulous to be angry. "Can't I just take that part off then?" I asked, trying to untie the scarf myself. But it was sewn on.

"Sorry, miss," the counselor said, not sounding sorry at all.

"Whatever. It's fine," I said, handing the stuffed animal back to Than and thinking that it had to be the dumbest application ever of an inconsistent rule. I was sure the long plastic strings that Fiona handed out earlier could do ten times the damage than my stuffed animal's five-inch *sewn-on* scarf. But what did I know?

"I'll see you tomorrow," Than said, giving me a hug.

Then he was escorted out, past the locked doors, and back into a free America.

I walked back to my room with Mia, who had a rotating circus of family and friends visiting her.

"That was weird, huh?" I said to her.

"Yep."

The same woman from earlier was lapping the halls, the one Billie said was named Gertrude, and Mia and I split our tandem to let her pass.

"You get clothes?" Mia asked, nodding at my bag.

"Yeah, you too, I'm guessing," I responded, noticing hers. "I've got books too. Let me know if you want to borrow one."

"Sure. Same."

"Cool."

I liked Mia. Her energy. Her attitude. I wondered if, in some parallel universe, we were friends in normal life.

My room came up first so we parted and I settled in for the night. Some people were still hanging out in Dayroom A and their scattered banter seeped into my room. I felt no desire to continue socializing—too tired—so I read the backs of each book that Than had brought me. Soon, a nurse came by with the med cart and handed me a tiny plastic cup with a pea-green and navy capsule.

"What's this?" I asked.

"Cymbalta. Mackenzie didn't tell you?"

"She talked about maybe switching my meds. I usually take them in the morning though." I took the pill obediently, thinking I would have preferred to read about the potential side effects and interactions first. I had seen a thousand Cymbalta TV commercials ("Depression hurts. Cymbalta can help!") and wracked my brain for any information or statistics I might remember.

"Will I still take my sertraline in the morning?" I asked, thinking about how much the withdrawal symptoms had sucked that one time during my sophomore year of college I had been dumb enough to not take my meds for a week.

"Um," the nurse hesitated, looking up my records. "Mackenzie didn't put that in. Maybe you can ask her when she comes in next?"

"Sure," I said. I figured that would be the next day, or that at least there would be another prescribing physician I could talk to. I had forgotten my daily dose the Thursday I came in, so I was already on Day 2 of no sertraline, and withdrawal symptoms usually hit me around Day 3. But the way I saw it, this nurse did not know anything about me or my medical history, so there was no point in telling her all this.

Around 9:00 p.m., a counselor came by with snacks (orange juice and more Lorna Doone's), and I enjoyed mine while cracking the spine of one of Than's books, cursing the fact that I could not lean up against the wall from my bed.

Feeling a bit calmer, I let myself live in the fantasy world of Stardust until, bleary-eyed and distracted, I switched off the light, closed my door to two finger-widths ajar, and tried to relax. But I did not feel at all rejuvenated or rehabilitated. I tried hard not to think about booty shots, pills, and ways to asphyxiate.

I had officially endured one complete day in the loony bin. What a way to spend a Friday night!

But maybe a change in perspective could make it better. The

best Friday nights are often spent in new places, with friends, and doing memorable things. Technically, all three of those qualities had been met. I had even laughed a few times that day. How bad can a day be, really, if it includes laughter?

I had the other women of the ward to thank for that laughter. I guess that was one thing about the ward. We could say whatever we wanted around each other and, with professionals rarely there to overhear, there were no repercussions. It was rather freeing to know we could say the craziest shit on our minds and that it would still be accepted as a piece of social capital. We laughed a lot during group and during meals—whenever we were together in the dayrooms. We had to.

While I was around this crew, I was feeling *something* besides loneliness or emptiness. Perhaps acceptance.

Despite feeling very little societal pressure to hide my mental illness, I can admit to "faking it" often. It is so much simpler to plaster on a smile than struggle to explain the torment going on inside my mind. And I enjoy the positive contagion; when I smile, others smile too. And I liked the world most when it was smiling.

But here? All bets were off. Around the other patients, there was no reason to be an artificial or augmented version of myself. It was liberating.

As for all these things happening to us—there was nothing fake about that either. This place was all too real.

II

Force Concentration

9

Lauren

There must be a fire. Flames must have burned away the mattress underneath me, and I must be lying on the ground. That is why I am stifling hot and why everything is so hard. I need to move, get up now, *and get outside.*

This is how my brain, awakened in the middle of the night by restlessness, rationalized the unfamiliar bed beneath me. Seeing the narrow window and the door ajar to the hallway, I remembered where I was. My momentary panic returned to gloom.

I wondered what time it was—it was still pitch dark outside. I turned away from the window to try drifting back to sleep but the middle-of-the-night-mind-running had already begun.

I was in the hospital right now, but eventually I would have to leave. What real life implications would I have to deal with once I did?

When I had sent myself to the ER during my freshman year of college, there had been serious repercussions. Even though the ER refused to admit me and discharged me in the morning, I returned to a shitstorm of administrative box-

79

checking, thanks to an overly-involved Housing & Residential Life program that needed to cover its own ass. Under threat of getting kicked out of on-campus housing, I was required to sign a behavioral contract that stated, if I ever did anything to harm myself, I would immediately be removed from the dorms. Despite not knowing my familial situation and the fact that I was an adult, a senior H&RL director forced me to call my father and inform him of "my situation." Then, twice a week for a month, I had to meet with the dorm's residential director, a skinny twenty-six-year-old man-child with a bowl cut who was condescension personified.

Those organizational hurdles had pretty much ensured that, should I ever feel unsafe or at-risk again, I would certainly not be going to Housing & Residential Life for help.

My residential advisor, Lauren, had lived in the room next door to me. She was an eccentric theater major that was a year older than me and called everyone on our floor "her ducklings." A few days after I returned from the ER, she knocked on my door and gave me a meaningful hug.

"If you ever need to talk," Lauren had said, "I'm here to listen. Unofficially—just to listen."

And eventually, sensing she was an ally, I opened up to her. I told her about my first almost-attempt in high school and how I had written The Note and laid out The Pills. I told her the thing I was most ashamed of: that I had looked into my little brothers' and sister's big admiring eyes and said goodbye. Every single moment with them since then, I had told her tearfully, was a gift.

Lauren was one of the most empathetic people I knew, and we grew closer over my freshman year. Little by little, I learned about her own battles with depression. We confided in each other and talked about how some authority figures were incredibly considerate and accommodating whereas others felt merciless to the point of cruelty.

A few months later, Lauren broke down and self-harmed and was sent to the hospital. The same day she got back from the hospital, she was fired from her position as an RA and given a few hours to move out of the dorms. All of the eighth floor residents found this out after she had been removed from the premises. Housing & Residential Life forbade her from contacting us to tell us why.

In the wake of losing her job and her home, she spiraled further and attempted to kill herself.

The policies put in place were in total opposition to the behavior that school administration *should* have been encouraging, which is seeking help when students need it under no threat of punishment. We had been punished for being mentally ill and offered no opportunity for redemption. And the reasons given—to preserve the safe, "distraction-free" environment—did not correspond to the feelings of the community. The people themselves—other students, many professors—were supportive, understanding, and kind. But the policies were rigid.

This happens all over the country, especially on college campuses. Students who exhibit signs of mental illness or imbalance have been smeared into submission and manipulated by massive institutions who falsely claim to have their students' best interests at heart. Another friend who previously attended Rice University before transferring to the University of Minnesota wrote an op-ed titled "Rice Maintains Happiest Students Status by Ousting Unhappy Students."[1] There are so many stories of students at schools like Northwestern,

Princeton, and Yale being evicted from campus housing, or forced to take required leaves of absence, after documented signs of even minor mental instability.[2,3] In some cases, all a student did was use their university's Mental Health Services. While it may sound like that is "just what the doctor ordered," if you read firsthand accounts from many of these stories, you notice a trend: the amount of time taken to understand and listen to each student's situation is ludicrously short. Students lose their autonomy with disturbing speed, which suggests that these "solutions" are rarely about the students' needs for recovery. They are about optics.

Lauren fought like hell. In February 2014, almost a full year after she was fired, she filed a discrimination complaint against Housing and Residential Life with the Office for Civil Rights, a branch of the U.S. Department of Health & Human Services. She knew they were unlikely to hear her case—they only investigate complaints made within 180 days—but her anger and pain had left deep scars and she hoped they would make an exception. Later that year in May, she told me that she had found an employment lawyer in her area and was pursuing a case with them. She followed up with the head of Housing and Residential Life to inquire about what was being done to remedy the situation. I do not know if she ever heard back. Then, nearly three years after she had lost her job, we had this conversation:

1/30/16, 9:37 PM

So. I sorta want to become a lawyer and then send a nice fuck you to ▇▇ and ▇▇▇▇▇

Like hey bitches your treachery and cruel treatment of my friends inspired me to go to law and fuck shit up

Like hey thanks for causing me existential anguish now I eat people like you for breakfast and make triple your aalary

Lauren – move forward, not backward. Don't do anything for or in spite of them because they are small people that don't matter.

That being said, if you become a kickass lawyer that ever encounters them or people like them, fuck them up.

Absolutely. They are merely people from the past who gave me a spark that united the eventual flame that's leading me to consider exploring the wonderful world of law

They are but a footnote in the long story of my life

On March 20, 2017, Lauren died by suicide. I had not heard from her in six months and I can only imagine the pain she must have been in. She left behind a father, a brother, and a fiancé.

I remember meeting her fiancé before they were engaged. She had been in a sorority at the time, and since males were not allowed upstairs in the bedrooms, she had asked if they could spend the night on my futon. Instead, I gave them the keys and told them to have a magical night—there needed to be more love in the world, and she had been so excited to spend time with him.

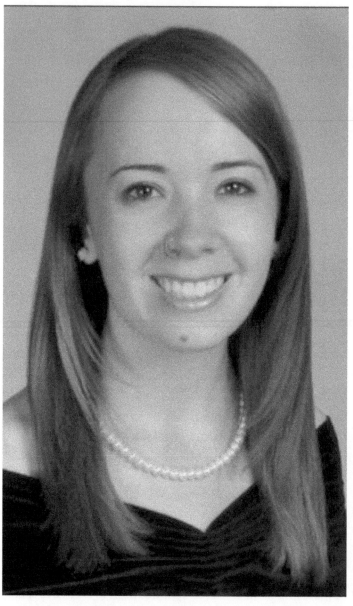

Lauren Erica Tank (1992-2017)

I remember when she told me she was adopting two orange kittens. "I want one to have a really majestic name," she said. "And the other to have a really derpy name." That's how she ended up with Ares and Kevin.

I remember when she responded with the kindest message when, on my birthday, I asked my Facebook friends to share a positive memory with me because I was feeling low. She mentioned the time in the first month of freshman year when I brought strawberries and Nutella around the dorm and said that's when she knew she would like me. She said she would love to see my face and hear my voice soon. And she told me I have a lovely soul.

I remember finding out she was gone. Katrina, a friend who had also lived on our floor freshman year, reached out to me to break the news. I stepped out of the meeting I had been in to talk to her and begin to process. Then I sobbed loudly in a bathroom corner at my client's office. I sent Lauren a message, "Why are you gone? Come back," knowing that she would never see it.

She would never see the outpouring of love that people showered her with on social media. She would never see the long, detailed memories that everyone shared on how she had positively impacted their lives. She would never see if any of it.

10

Decaf Coffee Still Makes You Shit

I wish I could reset the scene for you. Maybe add some rich descriptive verbiage about the setting, or reorient you to the changing circumstances. It would really bring you into the story. But the fact is, every moment in the ward was the same as the one before. Same drooling, shuffling patients. Same buzzing unfriendly lights. Same scuffed linoleum and same tired nurses scuffing the linoleum. And even though you have made it this far in, I cannot for the life of me imagine why you would want to feel like you were in there too.

I woke up at midnight, 2:00 a.m., and finally at 6:00 a.m. to Billie loudly advocating for someone. By that, I mean that she was getting into a heated debate with the counselor stationed just outside my room. I sighed into my pillow, trying to ignore their back-and-forth and wishing that I was allowed to just shut my door.

I finally peeked my head out and asked, "S'going on?"

"Oh, sorry, honey!" Billie said. "Didn't mean to wake you. Go back to sleep—it's still early."

But there was no point in trying to fall back asleep on my

gym mat of a mattress because, in a matter of minutes, an orderly was at my door to once again take my blood pressure. Soon afterward, people started doing their laps around the floor and asking about breakfast, which was still at least two hours away.

After an hour of tossing and turning, I gave up and turned back to my book. The story was fast-paced, fantastical, and easy to fall into. By the time the meal cart finally arrived, I was almost halfway through the story. I would need to ask Than to bring me books.

"Sleep okay?" Billie asked when I sat down next to her in the dayroom. "Sorry I woke you up so early."

"No worries. It's hard to sleep in here anyway. And I'll nap later. It's not like this coffee will do anything to keep me awake," I said, lifting up my plastic mug of decaf.

"I should probably still drink this crap," Nina was saying, biting into a French toast stick. "This food has me all blocked up. I haven't shit for days."

"Why does it have to be decaf," Angelique whined.

"Don't know, but it'll still make you shit," Nina grinned cheekily. She seemed less bubbly and bright today. If I had felt more conversational, I might have asked why.

In fact, most people seemed pretty run down. Mia hobbled in looking like a truck had hit her and told us that the Ambien she had been given the night before had been profoundly effective. "I feel like I could sleep for ten more days."

"Me too," Nina said. "They gave me Effexor and I'm gonna go back to bed after this."

Contrary to Mia and Nina, Brenda seemed to have a bit more pep. She was at least eating her breakfast with renewed energy but, like the rest of us, not talking much. We also had a new face at the table, Mary. She had short white hair, translucently pale skin, and the combination of her round glasses and the nearness of her eyes reminded me of a baby owl. She was eating applesauce like it was the best thing she had ever tasted. When I offered up my eggs to the room, she was the first to say, "Oh, me please."

I left most of my food on the tray, once again just picking out the pineapple and leaving the unripe melon, stale cereal, and dry French toast sticks to go back into the silver cart. This morning, I had a paper menu to fill out. I made my food selections with a dull crayon, circling "coffee" for all three meal columns, and then handed my menu back to the counselor on duty. Nurse Avery brought in the med cart and gave me my Cymbalta, now taken in the morning. Once again, I asked about any sertraline and whether a doctor would be in that day. I was told "I don't know" to both questions and so I just tossed back the capsule and the water she gave me without a fuss and then headed back to my room.

When I got there, Delilah's hulking figure was standing at the edge of my bed, hovering just above where my head would be if I had been in bed. The hairs on the back on my neck rose in apprehension.

"Um, Delilah?" I said uncertainly. "Can you get out of here?"

But she did not move. She smelled awful, like peppery mold. I switched to breathing through my mouth and asked again, "Delilah? Can you get out?"

The counselor outside heard me and barked, "Delilah! Get out of there! That isn't your room!"

"She's right next door; she's probably just confused," I explained, but the counselor did not acknowledge me and just yanked Delilah by the back of the gown until she lumbered out of my room.

Slightly shaken, I waved my hands around the air, trying to get the stench of body odor out. If I had woken up with her standing over me like that, I would have screamed bloody murder. And God, would the staff have even listened if I had tried to explain why I had screamed, or would they have just shot me in the ass with drugs until I was drooling on my stomach?

Trying not to imagine that scenario, I read a bit, walked around a bit, and closed my eyes to sleep a bit until a counselor walked through the halls announcing the next group therapy.

As I arose to get out of bed, I realized how off-kilter I felt. I recognized this particular brand of grogginess. The sertraline withdrawal symptoms were kicking in, starting with nausea. It was not quite the full-fledged vertigo that I knew would come eventually though, so I tried to ignore it and teetered toward the dayroom, hand lightly pressing on my stomach. On my way, I noticed Francine using her feet to scoot her wheelchair inch by inch toward the dayroom.

"Want me to push you in, Francine?" I asked.

She smiled her precious wide smile, showing me crooked teeth, and said, "Yes please, thank you."

I wheeled her in and dragged a heavy chair out of the way so she would have space at the main table. She thanked me again and then looked expectantly around the room.

Another Social Skills Group, I observed. Hoping it might be as exciting as yesterday's group with Sayed, I settled in, but neither Nina, Mia, nor Patty joined the group.

I sat between Francine and Angelique and listened politely to a woman named Karen tell us about Esteem. Her tone was warm, with none of the greater-than-thou airs that Sayed had given off during yesterday's session on good communication. Karen passed around two worksheets to each of us: the first, a three-columned list of words titled "Positive Traits," and the second, a complete-the-sentence page titled "About Me."

"So building good self-esteem can be done in a lot of ways," Karen told us all, "but I think an easy way to start is to think of some positive words that we think describe ourselves."

I skimmed the list. Words like *Strong* and *Brave* jumped out, as did less obvious ones such as *nurturing* and *mature*.

Karen passed around a Styrofoam cup of crayons and asked us each to go down the list, underlining all the words that we thought applied to us. "And this list is just the beginning," she added. "There are many, many more words like these, and if you get through the list and have extra time, go ahead and write down some more."

I took a green crayon and started at the top. Kind? I try to be. Intelligent? So I have been told. Hardworking? When the depression allows. I went through and found that I was underlining most of the words.

After we each took five minutes alone, Karen asked for volunteers to share the words they had underlined.

Francine went first. "I underlined 'em all," she said in her slight southern drawl. "And...and I think I have very good esteem." She smiled proudly, her shiny brown skin creasing wonderfully.

"That's fantastic," Karen encouraged. Then she turned to Mary. "What about you?"

"I circled a-a-all of them." Mary stuttered, but with confidence. "A-a-and I put a star next to 'Thoughtful' a-a-and I wrote down 'Smart' b-because I went back to school and got my GED."

"Wonderful," Karen said with a genuine smile. "That's an amazing accomplishment."

"Yeah," Mary agreed. "It was a great ac-accomplishment."

"What about you?"

Oh, she was talking to me. I looked down at my list, not wanting to read any of the words I had underlined. It would have felt boastful.

"I mean," I started hesitantly. Well, what the heck. "There was one word that I think describes me well that I didn't see on the sheet."

"Care to share?" Karen encouraged.

"Empathetic."

Francine asked, "What's that mean?"

I smiled at her. "It's like when you can imagine being in someone else's shoes and then you can express feelings about their situation better." When she smiled back uncertainly, I went on. "Like...remember just now in the hallway, how I helped wheel you into the room?"

"Yeah," she said.

"Well, I did that because I imagined being in the wheelchair myself, and knew that since my arms aren't very strong, it would be hard for me to get in here on my own. And I saw you having a hard time trying to scoot in with your feet, so I asked if you wanted help. Because if I was in your situation, I would have liked to get help too."

Francine's smile widened. "I think I'll write down that word t-too. How d'you spell it?"

I spelled out the letters and saw Karen nodding her appreciation to me. I nodded back. And though I did not put much effort into completing my "About Me" worksheet, I felt uplifted for the rest of the half-hour. It was the first therapy group that I saw value in for every attendee.

Later, when I was alone, I looked back at the words I had left untouched on the "Positive Traits" list. I had not underlined several: *Confident. Optimistic. Motivated. Funny. Patient. Modest. Serious. Independent. Trusting. Cheerful. Reliable. Relaxed. Listener. Decisive. Organized. Positive. Reasonable. Balanced.*

They were traits that I felt only applied to me at times when I was not feeling depressed or traits that felt entirely ingenuous or untrue. Some of them, like *optimistic* and *decisive*, were words that I could never see me using to describe myself since they were in direct contradiction to symptoms of my diagnosed mental illnesses.

Suddenly, I wanted to apologize for all the times when depression and anxiety had made me a bad friend, the times that I had been called a flake, or had come up short on a commitment because I had been too exhausted or too anxious to get myself out of the house. The sorrow and regret I felt, despite knowing that those feelings were not entirely fair, always compounded. At my most depressed and most anxious, I knew I was no fun to be around. It had to be something of a chore to have to include me, but my best friends were so intentional about never making me feel that way. All throughout college, my friends had been my superheroes—lifting my spirits, helping me battle villains, saving the day—and now the thought was occurring to me that I could never do enough to explain how much that meant.

In adulthood, that was even harder. The occasions to hang out required better planning and more intention. My friends and I all lived in different cities now, so airplanes had to be involved. With the stakes higher and my anxiety and depression only insignificantly improved, it was exhausting to make and maintain plans. One of the biggest motivating factors for keeping plans? I did not want *unreliable* to be one of my defining traits and I so hoped my friends knew that.

But that was not the only motivation. When I am surrounded by friends, it feels like I can do anything. It feels like I could be happy.

I knew, of course, that once I was discharged, I would tell all my friends from school and home and work about how I had spent my weekend. I owed it both to myself, to get the support I needed during the healing process to come, and to them, as a sign of my respect and trust. Knowing I was hospitalized and under observation might worry them, but I always figure it is best to be honest. That is how I have always shown my respect for relationships, both romantic and platonic. I want to be a truth-teller, honest to those around me, and, most important of all, honest to myself.

I turned back to the worksheet and neatly underlined *honest*.

Positive Traits

Kind	Insightful	Sensitive
Intelligent	Funny	Organized
Hardworking	Patient	Selfless
Loyal	Realistic	Practical
Attractive	Honest	Mature
Down-to-Earth	Generous	Focused
Goofy	Modest	Courteous
Creative	Serious	Grateful
Accepting	Independent	Open-Minded
Strong	Trusting	Positive
Friendly	Resilient	Responsible
Flexible	Cheerful	Cooperative
Nurturing	Self-Directed	Frugal
Thoughtful	Reliable	Tolerant
Confident	Relaxed	Innovative
Optimistic	Listener	Balanced
Respectful	Brave	
Determined	Decisive	
Skilled	Enthusiastic	
Helpful	Forgiving	
Motivated	Humble	

11

You Boat

I am about to serve you a long, gooey metaphor, so if that is not your thing, feel free to skip ahead. I promise that I will not be offended. It is not even an original metaphor—I am not trying to be original right now. I am trying to be frank.

I was in the psych ward for 106 hours. More than once, I caught myself trying to analyze what mini catastrophes and series of triggers had brought me there, but I could never identify the camel-back-breaking piece of straw. It was all of it—the full weight of life's cargo in the depths of my gut. The feeling of being alone in an endless ocean, not another ship or lighthouse in sight.

In life, I found staying afloat so tiring. I was lugging superfluous freight around, scared to let any of it go for fear it might turn out to be essential. Even my anchors, the spiritual or metaphysical things that typically stabilized me, felt heavy.

Then there was the ocean. Storms manifested out of nothing and angered the dark water into a frenzy. Mountainous waves threatened to topple me over. It was fight after epic fight with the elements.

Some days I thought about letting the ocean take me. I reasoned, would that really be *so bad*? To give up the fight, capsize, and let some of this heavy, heavy cargo fall away? For a moment, it would sound nice, to take a quick rest and let myself bob aimlessly for just a moment. Or I would imagine taking more drastic measures, like throwing my anchors overboard to just see where I drifted.

Then I would remember—I am a mighty ship. I was built to cut through seas and charge over the dark depths of the ocean unknown. Sinking means failure—I am no longer a ship if I sink. And abandoning my anchors means giving up any hope of one day resting in a safe, homey harbor.

Living with depression often feels like being a sinking vessel, but I can usually stop myself from thinking like that if I return to my purpose and identity. I was built to slice the sea. I was designed to displace the black bottomless water beneath me. That is what we do, as living things: We survive and we sail on.

So if I am a ship, and I am determined to continue staying afloat, something needs to be done about all of this sluggish-ness. Meds, exercise, eating healthy—these are all remedies that are like adding sails. They do not necessarily solve the problem, but they can help me move faster and be a better ship.

Another option is to throw extra baggage overboard. I compare this to mindfulness and meditation. Acceptance and exhalation. Knowing what is unnecessary and getting rid of it. This takes practice and a certain kind of strength, but there is no denying that it lifts some of the weight.

And then of course, the third option: remember I am not the only ship on the water. There are others, friends and loved ones, behind the fog, and their cargos may not be at capacity. They may be willing to help carry my load.

This option is my favorite. Find your fleet. Assemble your armada. Let them help you stay afloat. Because the physics of buoyancy is simple: the forces that lift you up just need to be greater than the forces that weigh you down.

12

Nice Weather Outside, Ladies

When I blinked awake from my mid-morning nap, my hands were shaking and glistening with sweat. As I turned to my side, waves of nausea hit me. My brain felt like it was being simultaneously squeezed and battered. Withdrawal symptoms were in full swing.

This could get bad. The one time I had stupidly gone an entire week without taking my meds, I became so disoriented with vertigo that I tumbled down half a flight of stairs and missed a day's worth of college classes.

Now what do I do, I thought. And again, I wondered when a doctor would come.

Unwilling to get up and risk reenacting my own version of Delilah and The Soup, I read my book from bed.

I would have skipped lunch to avoid moving, but I knew that someone would notice if my tray remained untouched in the silver cart, and I did not want anyone to record my absence in my chart—it could count against me. "Refuses food. Stays in bed. Recommend two additional days of psychiatric observation."

Even though it took ages for me to reach the dayroom with my tray, I was still one of the first ones there. Nina came in late, still quiet and somber. Mia came in even later, barely operational, trudging in her slippers. As a group, we could have passed for a horde of sluggish zombies.

"That Ambien they gave me last night..." Mia started, but she did not even bother to finish her sentence. She placed the elements of her lunch onto the communal table center and then shuffled back to her room. I did not see her again until after quiet hours.

Nina had been given an intense medical regimen that morning, and she was almost at Delilah's level of impassiveness. She was chewing slowly, and her eyelids drooped. The only person who seemed better today was Big Brenda, who, as with breakfast, was eating like a teenage boy who had hit puberty.

Right after lunch, Fiona was back with her craft cart. She had brought the newspaper, and I rifled through it for the crossword. Grabbing a crayon, I took a seat at the end of the table while the few women around me began to color sedately.

"Gorgeous weather today, ladies," Fiona chirped at us. "Isn't that lucky!"

We all ignored her—the nearest we could get to feeling the sun's natural warmth was pressing our foreheads against a south-facing window pane.

"Ninety-two degrees!" Fiona went on cheekily. "It might even be a bit *too* hot."

"Fuck off, Fiona," Billie said, a little too loudly.

I looked up to see if Fiona would react, but she either decided to pretend not to hear or realized what an insensitive thing that had been to say to a bunch of women who had no access to fresh air. Billie had not been outside in almost two weeks.

Fiona's sunny deportment in contrast to everyone else's sullen mood intensified the pit in my stomach—or perhaps that was the withdrawal. I left, holding the page of the newspaper against my stomach. I flopped back on my bed, not even bothering to attempt reading, and tried to meditate, tried to sleep, tried to do anything to get my mind off the dizziness and shakiness and clamminess I was feeling from lack of sertraline.

I must have drifted off at some point, because I realized the shadows in my room had all changed and that I was drenched in sweat. I probably smelled, and my teeth felt fuzzy. Cleaning myself off would surely make me feel better.

With my room's door still ajar, and the bathroom "door" nothing but a curtain, I stripped my clothes off and stood in front of the scratched-up mirror, unimpressed. That bit of me was eh. That part was okay. I liked that curve, that section of my skin, but hated the way I looked right there, there, and there.

Meanwhile, I twisted the shower knob all the way around, hoping that a bit of scalding water would relieve some of my tension, and then continued evaluating my naked body. Do all people do this? And does anyone ever like what they see?

I have, by all accounts, a just-fine figure. My stomach is flattish; I have abs when I flex. Men who have seen me naked have complimented my breasts. My navel goes in, and I have dimples on my lower back. But then there are the parts of me that I think are too small, too big, too round, not round enough. Sometimes I feel that way about my personality: in some places, too much. In others, too little.

As I looked at myself, I realized the bathroom mirror was not fogging up. *Shit.* I felt the water coming out of the nozzle and then tugged my hand back reflexively. Cold. *Shit shit shit.*

When I spent three weeks in rural Ghana, I bathed with a bucket of cold water and a bar of soap every day. That is fine, even preferred, when it is a hundred degrees and humid. But when you are away from home, locked in the over-air-conditioned psychiatric ward of a hospital, already frustrated, and exhausted from lack of sleep? *Then* it is not fine. It is all relative, of course, but under these circumstances, a cold shower might have been the most miserable thing possible.

During my entire stint on the fifteenth floor, I cried a fair amount, almost always out of sight. Realizing I would not be able to take a hot shower was the first time. I wanted that hot shower so badly, just to feel human.

Utterly defeated, I started to pull my clothes back on, trying to stop the hot, fat tears from pouring out of my face. I would not sob. And I would not let anybody see me cry. That had been the advice Billie had given me: only cry in the shower, so they cannot see you and give you more days. I have cried in public more times than I can count, but I would keep it together as much as possible in here. My public presence never mattered much to my sense of ego, but in the ward, it was not about pride—it was about freedom.

So I just stood on the grey tiles of the bathroom, half-dressed, rinsing myself off with a wet washcloth and soap. Screw the hair—I was not trying to look good for anyone in here.

When I finally calmed down, and after checking my face for splotchy redness or any other evidence of tears, I stood at my window and stared dolefully at the cityscape below. Some boys were skateboarding in the park at the base of my prison. They rolled from one end of the yard to the other, occasionally doing tricks before a recording iPhone. They were clearly enjoying the good weather, and I was glad for them. I could feel the sun on my face and wished I could be out there too.

As I stared through the window, a brown spider crawled across the inside of the glass pane. It was small, smaller than any of the beads in the bead bucket from group therapy, with stocky little legs. Robotically, I took my thumb and pressed against it, hard, until it was dead. I wiped my fingertip on the wall and then I returned to observing the ball-capped teenagers.

Normally I would have whimpered until one of my room-mates killed the spider for me, or I would have trapped it with a cup until someone else escorted it back into the wild, but today, with one purposeful touch, it was dead by my hand. I killed it just because I could. And the list of things I had the agency to do was getting shorter and shorter.

I was still feeling groggy. I was still sweating. My hands were shaking, and I did not feel like socializing (not that there were any group sessions to socialize during anyway). Instead I spent the afternoon rotating through all of my solitary activities, like a toddler in a room full of already-exhausted toys. I filled in some crossword clues with crayon but soon got frustrated and moved on. I sped through the Neil Gaiman book while hunched over on my bed. I dealt out and subsequently lost ten games of solitaire. And I even completed two mindless word searches from Fiona's pile of worksheets. My brain felt warped and unstimulated, soaking in the wrong balance of drugs while rotting on the vine.

The sound of the radio seeped out of Dayroom A and, bored of my activities, I plodded over to find Nina, Francine, and Angelique beading placidly. Nina still wore her bead crown around her head.

Whenever the radio played, a nurse or counselor had to unlock the closet, set a station and volume level, and then relock it. Whoever had requested music had chosen a classic rock and pop channel; the tunes were muted but discernible behind the heavy closet door.

"Fiona left the beads out for us," Angelique said in welcome.

"That was nice of her," I said, taking a seat and rummaging through the printables left behind. "Let's be sure not to choke on them to thank her for her unsupervised kindness." I chose a picture of potted flowers and grabbed a few crayons.

"Her and Billie really got into it," Nina said, her voice still slurring a bit.

"Yeah, but still. Fiona brought her iced coffee this morning," Angelique said, with clear envy in her voice. "*Real coffee.*"

"She was just sucking up to Billie, because she knows who really runs this show," smiled Nina. As the song changed, she closed her eyes and turned her face to the ceiling. "Ahh. Pink Floyd."

"Where *is* Billie," I asked.

"She doesn't like being in here when there's music and talking at the same time," Angelique explained. "Because of her ear."

"I bet she tells that iced coffee story really well," I commented.

"You okay, hon?" Nina asked me, seeing my hands tremble on the table. "They got you fucked up on something?"

"Nah, the opposite. That girl Mackenzie changed my meds yesterday but I was on a high dosage of sertraline and yeah…" I shrugged. "Withdrawal." I felt stupid bringing up withdrawal to Nina since I knew she had gotten clean from heavy heroin use five years ago, and the symptoms I was feeling now were nothing compared to that.

But instead of judging me, she grimaced sympathetically. "They don't know what they're doing here. They put me on Effexor this morning and I just feel *fucked up*."

"You don't need the drugs," Angelique said.

"I really don't," Nina agreed. "I'm way better without them. They talk to me for five minutes and then decide that I need them now. It's fucked."

"It is," I agreed.

We sat listening to the music, bobbing our heads and appreciating the peace. Eventually "Happy" by Pharrell Williams came on. I closed my eyes and was back in the summer of 2014, dancing to cheesy choreography on the Baltic Sea. Then Justin Timberlake's "Can't Stop The Feeling" played, and I was once again behind the lens of a camera filming the most joyous music video of children that anyone has ever seen.

Music is such a gift. The right song can trigger the perfect memory and transport you to a brighter place. Feelings that seemed unreachable can once again be felt with the right track. Music can connect us across cultures, languages, backgrounds, and states of mind—even songs as overplayed as the ones I was hearing now. And it is a great mood-manipulator. I have spent countless evenings exploring the boulevards of Chicago with my headphones. In my experience, there are very few cloudy moods that cannot be sunnied with a long walk and a good playlist.

In the dayroom, everyone bobbed their heads and mouthed the lyrics they knew. Francine sang, though her singing sounded more like a chant.

"Think they'd let us stay in here for quiet hours?" Angelique asked, her fingers running over a plate of beads.

Her innocent question was met with scoffs from around the table. "No way," Nina said definitively.

My stomach flip-flopped from nausea, and I suddenly wanted to be away from the music. This was not *my* music. It was just one more thing I had no control over, and one more stimulant to increase my queasiness. I grabbed a red, purple, and orange crayon, my barely-touched flower picture, and excused myself from my friends. Even when I got to my room, though, I felt unsettled.

I wanted to be outside. I wanted to go home and enjoy the summer weather. I wanted to be biking on the boulevards, listening to my *own* playlist. Maybe get an Italian ice from Miko's or just climb out the window of my apartment and read on the back roof. The sun just looked so *nice* outside, and I wanted to feel its warmth directly on my face—not through a glass window.

Sighing, I grabbed my incomplete crossword and went out into the hall. It was almost quiet hours. Might as well start early.

Fiona was on hall duty, and I went up to her with newspaper in hand. "I know you can't let me have a pen," I started sweetly, "but if I sit right here next to you, and you can watch me, can I just borrow it so I can do the crossword?"

She looked at me and must have decided that I seemed harmless enough. "You'll stay right here?"

"Right here," I promised.

She passed her pen to me, and I sat cross-legged next to the water fountain, triumphant. Writing with a pen again was glorious. The black ink seeped into the page, making my lines clear and defined. Admiring the straight, bold letters I could now create, I filled out as many clues as possible. I bobbled my head from side-to-side like a kid, hoping Fiona would notice how happy this simple thing made me. Quiet hours were announced, and those in the dayroom filed back into their rooms.

A few minutes later, Counselor Andrej approached Fiona to relieve her of hallway duty. The Changing of the Guard. He noticed me sitting there and out of the corner of my eye, I saw him jab his thumb at me and raise his eyebrow at Fiona.

"I told her she could use my pen for her crossword as long as she stayed there," Fiona said in response.

Andrej shifted his weight awkwardly and then spoke to me. "It's quiet hours now, though."

"I know," I said confusedly. "I'm being quiet."

"But you need to go back to your room."

"My room's *right there*," I said softly, pointing not five feet away across the hall.

He gave Fiona a look of blame and then back down at me. "I really need you to go back to your room now."

"Why?" I challenged, still trying to act sweet and innocent but starting to get irked. Was this such a big deal?

"I just—" and then he put his hands on his hips. "I don't want the other ones to get jealous!"

I raised my eyebrows calculatedly. "Jealous?"

"Yeah," he forged on. "Because you get to be out in the hallway and they can't."

I looked at the otherwise empty hallway and then at Fiona, hoping she would step in and say that there was really no harm being done.

Andrej continued, "And besides. You're not supposed to have a pen anyway."

I knew I would not win. I folded up my crossword, stood, then placed the pen slowly back on the guard desk, all without breaking eye contact. Andrej was the first to look away.

Coward.

I could feel Fiona's apologetic grimace follow me as I returned to my room. I shut the door firmly enough for Andrej to hear the soft *click* and relished in the fact that if he wanted to reopen it, he would have to get his ass off the seat he had just settled into.

Back to square one. I flopped onto my bed, on my stomach, and turned to look at the window. Looking straight out, my fifteenth floor view was dull, just three vertical rectangles. Rough concrete on the left. Blue sky in the middle. Faded yellow curtain on the right. *I could paint that*, I thought, *and no one would know what a miserable painting it really is.*

My thoughts were everywhere and nowhere. I wanted to be in that beautiful blue rectangle, part of that sunshine, and shaded by those clouds. I wanted to feel softness, not stiff bedsheets. I wanted to smell anything besides antiseptic, denial, sadness, and soaped-over piss.

My mouth was dry but I was too stubborn to walk across Andrej's hall to the water fountain. My feet were hot but taking my socks off and exposing skin to these dusty floors was not an option. My hands were still clammy. My head was starting to pound. I wanted to scream and sob and stand on my bed to punch the ceiling tiles. I wanted a pen and my stuffed penguin and a strawberry-banana smoothie.

Mostly, right now, I wanted to slap Andrej across the face for denying me something as simple as a pen.

Cracking open Than's book, I tried to immerse myself in fantasy, but even *Stardust* failed me as a distraction; the final pages came up before quiet hours were even halfway over. I finished coloring the flower petals and then used more Vaseline to paste it to the window. Just as I was looking around the room for something else to occupy my time, thinking exasperatedly how long an hour really was, I heard one of the heavy hallway fire doors slam.

13

Caged

Pressing my ear to the door, I heard large socked feet shuffling outside my room.

Then quiet.

Then more shuffling.

I cracked the door a centimeter and peeked out but could see nothing besides two counselors, one of them Andrej, standing like bouncers on either side of the southwest fire doors. I pulled my door open more, knowing they would not be able to see me unless I stuck my head out, and glanced furtively around the other hall for the source of the shuffling.

It was the pregnant-but-not-pregnant girl. She was peering around the corner just across from me, looking absolutely terrified. She did not seem to see me, or at least did nothing to acknowledge I was there.

"Greta, we need you to get back in your room," the other counselor said in a bored tone.

But how was she supposed to do that without getting past them? They had locked the doors, and her room was on the other side.

"Greta, come here, please," Andrej said.

They could not see her expression, but I could. She looked like a gigantic caged animal coming to the realization that she was trapped. Her face was white, eyes bulging, about to cry. She looked truly pathetic, in her hospital pants and purple tank top that left most of her arms and torso uncovered. She shuffled down the hall to the locked doors and tried the handle to no avail.

I heard the counselors mutter to each other and then walk closer toward me, toward Greta, boxing her in even more. I shut my door before they walked past, knowing what was about to happen.

Greta's wail filled the air just as they turned the corner. Her cries and shouts of "No! Stay away from me!" got louder and more desperate. I knew they would be pinning her down, giving her a shot, even though all they would have had to do, it seemed, was open the door and shepherd her back to her room. I imagined that Billie would be poking her head out by now and watching the scene, tears in her eyes.

I backed deeper into my room, hands over my ears, trying to drown out Greta's weakening yells and the voices of other patients now adding to the commotion. I wanted to scream to the counselors, "Get your hands off her!" but I also wanted to go home. So instead, I cried silently to myself on the tiled floor behind my shower curtain, so very, very ashamed of doing nothing.

14

Unfuck The World

Our squad had developed psych ward lingo, used only by the tight-knit bunch of us and mostly serving to describe other patients. Cats, short for catatonic, referred to those patients who just stayed in their beds all day or moved at a sloth's pace to sit unblinkingly in the dayrooms. Then there were Kittens, patients like Mary, who were harmless and simple-minded. And then there were Ferals. You did *not* want to engage with a feral.

Greta was not a cat, and she was not a Kitten, and she was not violent or unreasonable enough to be a Feral. And she was not one of *us*, although she could have been if she wanted. Even in this museum of misfits, not everyone had a place.

After quiet hours were over, many folks went back into the dayroom in order to gossip about the quiet hours showdown. Others went to continue their art projects or just get out of their lonely cells. We learned that Old Brenda and Carla were getting discharged, and we passed judgment on why they should get to leave when both were practically Cats. Unlike their animal counterpart, psych ward Cats were not equipped to take care of themselves.

"She's been here less than I have," Nina was saying enviously of Carla, "and I'm doing way better than she is."

"Yeah, but what insurance do you have?" Billie pointed out. "They probably know they can get more money out of you, but not her."

"Yeah, they're both Medicaid," Big Brenda said.

"Figures," Billie said critically. "It's all about the money, isn't it."

"You really think?" I asked, not wanting to believe.

"Got a better explanation?" Billie retorted.

Little Brenda was back with us. She was hugging her knees, looking grumpy and annoyed. "Why did I come here?" she huffed. "I should have just gone to a spa."

"That certainly would have been cheaper," I said.

"And probably more effective," Mia agreed, and then she sighed, "God, let's all go to a spa."

Carla chimed in suddenly from her seat at the end of the room. "I'll go to the spa for all of us!"

Mia rolled her eyes but had to smile. "Thanks, Carla."

"I just want to go home," Angelique admitted.

"You will," Nina comforted. "We all will—eventually."

Then the conversation shifted to a discussion on what we missed about being home. Mia missed coffee (and her boyfriend), Angelique missed her cat (and her boyfriend), and Nina missed having sex (with her boyfriend).

"I saw your boyfriend when he visited yesterday, Mia," Billie said. "He was a cutie."

Mia made a face.

"I wish my boyfriend could visit me," Angelique said. "But he isn't eighteen yet so they don't let him."

"Oooh," Nina teased. "You're dating a younger man!"

Angelique blushed and kept her eyes trained on her beads. "Whatever!"

"I miss my bed," I said. "It's like a cloud. And I sleep in the same spot every night so it kind of sinks into a little nest now. And I wish I could sleep there instead of on these stupid mattresses." I put air quotes around the word "mattresses" and buried my face in my arms.

"It'll happen," Nina said. "You're so sweet to all the nurses and everyone. Your doctor will let you out soon."

"I haven't even seen a doctor yet," I whined. "Do we know when one's coming?"

"They'll come when they come, that's all I ever get told," Billie replied.

"Incredible," I said sarcastically.

"It's so fucked up," said Mia. "We're in a hospital. Shouldn't there be doctors, like, all the time?"

Billie let out a dry laugh. "You'd certainly think so!"

"Like seriously, they just put us on meds, and no one's even checking!" Mia's voice started to rise and I eyed the door as she went on, "I want a list of everything I'm on. And what side effects they have! So I can show my uncle later."

"Good luck getting that," I said.

"I'm gonna ask." And she marched off toward the nurse's station. *Action-oriented*, I thought. I liked that.

"Good for her," Billie said as Mia's ponytail disappeared around the corner.

Not wanting to color or bead or do another freaking word search, I busied myself by taking a closer look at all the artwork taped up around the room.

The art was just as colorful and varied as its wonderfully

psychotic patients. In a glass display case next to the window, there was a series of collages, created during a time when there must have been women's magazines and glue sticks available. There was one piece covered in purple with cut-outs of Prince that read, "for Fiona." Papers of varying sheens were layered thickly, barely contained behind the glass, with all lengths of inspirational messages written in capital letters. Flowers, hearts, peace signs, and stick people were the common motifs, a true garden of medicated hippie wisdom.

After the display case had been filled, featured colored-in printables had been taped around it. In the past, there must have been construction paper, oil pastels, higher-quality crayons, and glitter—materials that shone and popped off of the yellowing walls.

One of my favorites had a rainbow and read, "For real I love the Lord. But here the bible is deemed contraband." I had to chuckle because I could just imagine somebody bringing in their hardcover copy of the bible, only to have staff members tell them that no, hardcovers were not allowed and that it would have to stay locked in the contraband closet but they could wait for a chaplain to stop by with a paperback version but oh, that could be awhile.

Billie noticed me inspecting the art and sidled up to me to add her commentary. "Did you see what we put in the window earlier?"

I shook my head, already grinning. "Show me?"

She ushered me to the other window where seven of Fiona's printouts had been heavily colored in with black or purple crayon and stuck to the window.

"We put a message on the back," Billie said, barely able to contain her glee.

I squinted to look past the thick layer of crayon wax that was filling in the cartoon animals and flowers. With the afternoon sun streaming in from behind, I could just barely eke out the letters on the back: *H-E-L-P U-S-!*

"Amazing," I said. Even from fifteen floors away, I bet some people on the sidewalk were getting a chuckle.

"This one too," Billie said proudly, pointing at a picture of a rooster she had shoved into the frame of a Patient Rights poster. In black crayon, she had scribbled, *do u like my cock?*

I opened my mouth at her. "They're gonna be so pissed!"

But Billie shrugged, unfazed. "I used to write only positive messages, but then they didn't like those either. Like this one," and she started walking toward the door, "that I had up until Fiona threw it in the garbage."

She unstuck the door from its magnetic stopper and showed me the crumpled poster she had fished from the trash. "UN-FUCK THE WORLD," it read boldly.

"I like it," I told her matter-of-factly.

"Yeah," Billie replied. "So now it's back here, where she'll never find it."

We both stared at it awhile before Billie added, "Don't know what her deal with it was."

I grinned and gave Billie a one-armed hug. "I know right? Really, it's a positive message."

I did love it. The poster was intrepid, unapologetic, and rooted in good sentiment—just like Billie. And the message was on point, really: No matter on what scale, we should all be reminded to make some piece of the world a better place.

I made a mental note to make "UNFUCK THE WORLD" a new mantra. I typically have a good saying in my mental back pocket, something to quell the internal cyclic ramblings.

Whenever my anxiety gets bad, and I am in a situation where I need to Hold It Together, I repeat one of my mantras to myself. No one is any the wiser, and I can deal with my worries in anxious peace.

But anxiety does not just mean worrying about everything. That is an oversimplification. It is also overthinking and being unable to drown out your own self-doubting voice. It is muscle tension and insomnia and chest pain. And the second-third-and-fourth-guessing—there is no end. The distinction between what is logic and what is anxiety can be so fuzzy; I do not know what my own inner voice sounds like without the apprehensive tone and lilt of insecurities woven in.

I am no authority on anxiety, but here is how mine typically works. Every day is a hundred little battles, a hundred pieces of straw. And sometimes I am fifty straws away from back-breakage and sometimes I am just five. But everything is a straw, from making my coffee order smoothly in a busy Starbucks line, to succinctly giving my updates at a work meeting and making a clever joke with friends. Everything is more difficult, and the stakes are always, always high.

You know how in movies when a character is making decisions, a little devil—poof!—appears on one shoulder and a little angel—poof!—appears on the other, and they will talk back and forth about what their protagonist should do? Well, imagine anxiety as Winnie-the-Pooh's friend Piglet, just stuck in the middle in the little crevice of your collarbone, wringing his little hands and saying, "Oh d-d-d-dear."

That's anxiety. A little Piglet who hangs out around your throat.

It took years before I realized that other brains did not work like this—at least, not to this degree. My depression was a little easier for me to identify because it came in waves, and I knew how it felt when it was "off" (or, better put, "less-on").

But my anxiety was constant. Sometimes it was a breeze blowing against me, annoying but ignorable, and sometimes it was a run-for-cover hurricane. When the evacuate-immediately-it's-a-natural-disaster level episodes became too frequent, I realized not everyone reacted to stress like I did, even among my high-performing high school peers. Not everyone needed to take a three-hour nap after a long day at school, and not everyone was so preoccupied with worry that they forgot to eat meals. Certainly, most of my AP classmates were not crying before every single test.

When it first began to dawn on me that anxiety would be something that I would have to deal with for a long time, I was convinced that it would prevent me from Being Successful. That fear was coupled with depression too—how could I possibly get anywhere in life when I was so exhausted from battling myself? And even if I Became Successful, that was certainly no guarantee of long-term health and happiness. The two were almost unrelated. Plenty of successful people—celebrities, business tycoons, you name it—still succumbed to their pain.

Ned Vizzini was one. He authored the young adult novel *It's Kind of a Funny Story* based upon his own experience being hospitalized for suicidal depression at age twenty-three. I read his book sometime in middle school and loved it for it frankness, unique characters and quirks. In 2010, when the book was made into a movie with Zac Galifinakis, I saw it and loved that too. Despite Vizzini converting his pain into a beautiful and well-loved story, he was still unwell. He used his ongoing anxious energy as fuel for publishing other novels and launching a successful Hollywood writing career. He continued to have lows, and one of those lows, his wife said, he did not come out from. At thirty-two years old, as a bona fide success, he jumped off the roof of his parents' Brooklyn building and died.

I knew, even if I came out of this hospital experience on the other side, my long-term mental health was still up in the air. I wanted to get there, to be healthy. But sometimes I did not know which illness to tackle first: depression or anxiety. Perhaps it was not wise to separate the two since they could be so intertwined, and each often exacerbated the other.

Still, they were very different beasts, and taking on two beasts at once—well, I am just not that skilled of a huntress.

15

I Need No Sympathy

It is hard to make bad spaghetti. In regular life, I made it for myself all the time, once a week at my most frequent. I do nothing fancy—just boxed vermicelli, some ground beef browned up over the stove, and half a jar of Prego or Ragu or Newman's Own, depending on the sales. I will add fresh garlic if I remembered to buy it, or chop up whatever vegetables I have left from making tacos. Ten minutes at the stove and I have a hot and filling meal with plenty of reheatable leftovers. It's easy, reliable comfort food. It nourishes.

I think that is why I was so disappointed when I tasted the first bite of the spaghetti on my dinner tray. It was not just cold, it was flavorless! The noodles tasted strange and had a weird rubbery texture that I did not know you could get from pasta—wasn't it either undercooked and al dente or overcooked and mushy? And I would have bet my visiting privileges that the sauce they used was "meat flavored" instead of containing any actual meat. Those chunks in the sauce could have been anything.

I sighed and started adding milk and sugar to my decaf.

"What the fuck is wrong with those idiots in the kitchen?" Mia was saying ruefully, staring in dismay at her plate. "Do they not know what '*vegetarian*' means?"

I looked down at the pale salad in front of her. Not only did it look disgusting—there was more white than green on that lettuce, and the sprinkled cheddar cheese was sweating—but there were clearly cubes of ham and bacon bits throughout the entire thing.

On the bright side, at least Mia had gotten her attitude back. It was a relief; seeing her strung out on whatever cocktail of meds the staff had put her on had been depressing. Nina was almost back to normal too and she was poking a fork through Mia's salad.

"Yeah, that's inedible," Nina concluded. "Here, want some of my..." and she looked down her own tray for anything vegetarian and substantial, but came up empty. "Yeah, I got nothin'. Sorry."

Mia let out a sound of frustration and started picking at the fruit cup on her plate.

"I didn't get cake like the rest of you," I complained.

"You didn't?" Big Brenda mumbled, mouth full.

"At least you got silverware," Angelique said, looking around her tray and the rest of the table for a plastic fork. Angelique's trays were always missing something vital. Since she was marked as a "self-harm watch," she was not technically allowed to have a plastic tray, since that could *obviously* be used as a weapon. Instead, she was supposed to receive her meals on a Styrofoam tray, but the kitchen always just put her Styrofoam tray on top of the normal plastic one, because of course.

Mia pushed her tiny cake plate toward me, saying, "I don't

want it. It probably tastes terrible though."

"Yeah, probably. Thanks."

The usual swapping and groans over what had been missed or mistaken went on. I forced a few spoonful's of the spaghetti down and then moved on to Mia's chocolate cake, which tasted more like a slightly stale cake donut than actual cake but was quite edible between swigs of coffee. I was in a better mood; right before dinner, I had spoken to Than on the phone, and he had told me that my friend Faith was going to visit that night too. I also conveyed my wishlist for the day: my glasses, more books, and a pad of paper, but no hardcovers or staples. He promised to bring everything and to be there at 6:30 p.m. sharp.

On top of that, Billie had slipped me a turquoise marker just before we had sat down to eat. "For your crosswords. Hide it in your sleeve. Don't get caught with it!"

We were psych ward smugglers, and it was kind of fun.

Even though the meal had tasted terrible, having that many carbs in my stomach did at least help with my nausea and vertigo. After we all finished eating, we stuck around to listen to the radio, the sound leaking out from underneath the closet door. It was still tuned to the same pop-rock station from before. Familiar chords began, and suddenly we looked up at each other, grinning giddily. The opening lines of "Bohemian Rhapsody" filled the room and we transformed.

"Ready?" our faces asked each other. Some of us already had our eyes closed and were mouthing along. And at first, we sang melodically, barely attracting the attention of anyone in the hall and miming the actions in the song. The music swelled into its crescendos and our singing grew louder.

Caught in a landslide / No escape from reality

I gesticulated dramatically. Mia bobbed her head with her face toward the ceiling. Nina crooned. Even Angelique, at nineteen, knew most of the words.

Easy come / Easy go / Little high / Little low

We were all poor boys, all mamas, singing to each other and telling each other to carry on as if nothing really matters. We swayed. We sang. We pretended to shred on imaginary guitars. And when the song shifted to the theatrical turn, we contorted our faces and sang all the parts, loudly, until the Kittens at the other tables in the room were clapping along gleefully.

Bismillah! / We will not let you go / LET HIM GO!

I wanted to jump onto the table, kick all the dinner trays, stomp out "*Never, never, never, let me go!*" I wanted to really get crazy because it was freakin' "Bohemian Rhapsody," and why not, we were already in the crazy coop.

In the music video version of this memory, all of the orderlies and nurses burst in wearing riot gear, and it is patients versus staff, with dinner trays and heavy chairs as our weapons. An all-out food fight breaks out in Dayroom A, with dramatic slow-motion shots of spaghetti splattering in Andrej's face, coffee staining Fiona's shirt, Sayed slipping on the linoleum and faceplanting into Mia's ham salad. Our hospital gowns flap wildly like capes, and the Kittens jump and clap for us. It's me, Nina, Billie, Angelique, Patty, Mia, Big Brenda, and Delilah, all holding hands and racing out to the rest of the ward to bang on everyone else's door so they can join the fight.

So you think you can stone me and spit in my e-e-eye / So you think you can love me and leave me to die-e-e?

We outnumber the staff four-to-one and now it is a full-on brawl. The camera gets shots of syringes squirting clear liquid into the air, pills flying everywhere as staff are tripped and tied up so that we can continue our rampage. Someone finds the keys, and we bust onto the other adult behavioral floors. Men from the floor below join us. Then teens. It's a magnificent madhouse.

Just gotta get out / Just gotta get right out of he-e-ere

And we all tumble down fifteen flights of stairs, most of us barefooted. We crash through the stairwell doors onto the main street and then the world returns to normal speed. Bystanders on the street stop and gawk at us, and some whip out their cellphones to start live streaming the scene. In public, we feel ridiculous. We all turn around dejectedly and file back up the stairs.

Nothing really matters / Anyone can see

We each return to our designated rooms. The staff, dumbfounded, bring us our Ativan doses, which we complacently swallow. Final scene: someone reciting to Caroline, "*Nothing really matters / to me,*" with a blank stare. They lie on their side in their psych ward bed.

Any way the wind blows

Fade to black.

16

Goodnight Crazies Everywhere

One of the worst parts of depression is how quickly great moments can be swallowed up and overtaken by the returning darkness. It was just a song, but for the five minutes it played I had been free and flying. But as it finished, the high was immediately tempered by the all-consuming pain, so familiar that I might have mistaken it for comfort.

I thought back to Thursday night—was it really just two nights ago?—when Dr. Patel was asking me questions about my mental state. He had asked if I was suicidal, and I had paused. But no, I was not suicidal. I didn't know if had ever been suicidal because I didn't think that I had ever wanted to commit suicide. Hold on, let me repeat that to myself to see if it tastes true.

I have never wanted to kill myself.

Truth.

But I *have* been in so much pain that I thought about dying. And I think there is an important distinction there. Having suicidal thoughts is not the same as being suicidal. At least, that is what makes sense to me. Sometimes, as a means of escape, I might daydream about what life around me would be like if one day I was not there. When I am at my lowest, it seems better. Less burden on my friends. Less children to keep tabs on. And I wish I knew how to mute those kinds of thoughts but they can be so strong. And it is a strange type of release to imagine how life could go on without you. Some of the weight is lifted off and, for a moment, it feels a little easier to breathe.

There was a time in my life when the first thing I would do when I entered a room was scan for all the ways I could kill myself. Those electrical outlets there, plus my metal hair clip. That extension cord hanging from that hook. A plastic bag. Anything sharp. All within a second of crossing the threshold. But I did not *really* want to die, even at my lowest. Rather, it was like being claustrophobic, and finding comfort in knowing where the exits were in case of an emergency. And locating the "exits" made it a little easier for me to act normal, a little easier to breathe. Does that make sense?

Other times, my suicidal thoughts manifested as ambivalence toward my own safety. Small things, like not wearing a seatbelt or only looking one way at a busy intersection. Even then, I did not want to die. But I didn't *not* want to die. I didn't really care either way.

Even when I am feeling stable and healthy, the intrusive thoughts of suicide are there, clamoring in the back of my skull. Images of my grieving family, or my things being boxed up by my friends, pop up in my dreams and then haunt me. How do you forget shit like that? How do you get that out of your mind? No therapist has been able to give me a foolproof way. It feels like there are no cures, just coping mechanisms. And even when I am well, my thoughts could still be sick.

The thing that keeps me from surrendering to the intrusive thoughts, and will always keep me alive, is knowing that dying would have consequences for those I love, those I love more than life—and more than death—itself. If I could cease to exist, just fade away as if I never was, that would be one thing. But to leave my little brothers and sister without their teammate, to leave my parents without their firstborn, to leave my friends and coworkers and neighbors and community with a hole in the fabric I have become part of? I just will not do that.

And so, when visiting hours started and I met Than in the hallway outside Dayroom B, I hugged him for longer than usual. And in hugging him, I hugged everyone else, and thanked them for existing and helping me exist, and making me smile and laugh and giving me reasons to cry.

"You good?" Than said, breaking the hug.

I nodded, eyes shining, and we went into the day room where a few others were settling into their visits too. I was wearing the giant turtleneck sweater he had brought me that made me look like Oscar the Grouch's gray cousin.

Than handed me the legal pad and the glasses (both checked for hidden weapons by Psych TSA). He had ripped out the used sections, leaving me about twenty pages, forty front-and-back, that I was excited to fill.

"Thanks," I said to Than, smiling easily. "I'm probably gonna fill this up."

"I'll bring another if you need it."

"How are you?" I asked. Then I asked if he had talked to our other roommate.

"Yeah," Than answered. "I talked to him."

"I don't think I'll call him," I told Than. "He won't know what to say. I don't want to make him feel bad for that."

Than shrugged and filled me in on who else had inquired. He also told me that he and his mom and done some light research on the hospital, "and this place is the lowest rated."

"Sounds about right," I muttered.

"When can you get out?"

I rolled my eyes. "Don't know. Still haven't seen a psychiatrist."

"Well, if you're not out by Thursday, Mom'll get you out," he assured me. Than's parents were visiting the upcoming weekend, something I was very excited for. Than's parents were the best, the type of parents I hoped to be. When I had been in Pittsburgh a few months prior for work, I had tried to take them out for dinner but when it came time to paying the check, Than's dad almost knocked a glass off the table in his effort to block my credit card from the waitress. "Old person's privilege," he had said.

"I'd love to see your mom take this place down," I said, chuckling.

Then I saw my friend Faith's apprehensive face pop out from around the corner. As soon as her eyes found me, her expression morphed into one of sympathetic concern, cautious joy, and so much love. As always, she looked perfectly polished, today in a hot pink chiffon top that was stylishly chic and somehow still professional. We had met at our first day of training at work and, with shared drives to achieve, compete, and excel, had bonded quickly. Seeing her made me grin, and I got up to hug her tightly because hugs are the best and I was so happy to see her, even if my face was oily and my hair was full of grease.

I sat down, looking at the pair of über-supportive friends in front of me, smiling foolishly. I was feeling hardly any withdrawal side effects now and I had over an hour with these two wonderful people.

Faith came with questions about the facility, and I answered them as best I could, with Than adding details from what he had read online whenever I took a breath. She widened her eyes dramatically when I told her I had not seen a doctor yet, and I chose then to leave out some of the more dramatic details, like booty shots and the uncaring staff. Instead, I told them about some of the funny signs in Dayroom A.

"And there's this gem in here," I said, pointing my thumb to the picture of the toilet that read, *YOU ARE NOT SHIT.* "I think that's my favorite one. Even more than 'the bible is deemed contraband.'"

"There's really no therapists around, though?" asked Faith, clarifying from one of my earlier statements.

"Just babysitters. Although, I'm not sure how useful therapists would be here. No one really listens to us. But it's okay, we talk with each other, and I guess that's our therapy."

"I'm glad you've met good people here," Faith said earnestly.

I pointed out some of the other folks in the room who had visitors. "That's Mia—we came in on the same day. She's awesome." I twisted around. "And that's Angelique. She's nineteen. She's awesome too."

I told them about how I had been staying busy, telling Than that I had finished the Neil Gaiman book and enjoyed it.

"And I still can't do the crossword in pen, although one person let me use hers as long as I stayed next to her."

"Why can't you use a pen?" Faith asked, shocked.

I mimed stabbing myself in the neck and then bleeding out in the table. She didn't know whether to laugh or look horrified, and her reaction ended up being a bit of both.

"It's fine though," I said, sitting up. "One of my friends snuck me a marker, which is ten times better than a crayon."

"They're that strict here, huh?" Faith asked incredulously.

"Oh yeah." I tried to keep my tone as light and nonchalant as possible.

The conversation shifted to them talking about real life, with Than listing off the errands he had run that day, and Faith updating me on the status of her project search at work. I listened, happy for the distraction, but all too soon it was 8:00 p.m., and they were being kicked out of the ward. Faith gave me another two-armed hug, telling me she would visit again on Monday, and she and Than walked through the locked door.

Mia's visitors left with them, leaving us to stare at each other with the same thought.

"We need to get out of here," she said to me.

"Yeah, we do."

As we walked toward Dayroom A, where the rest of our crew was passing time, she told me about another partial inpatient program that she had previously gone to, and how it compared. It sounded so much better, with supportive staff, personalized programming, and professional group therapies. Then she continued with how this place was doing more damage than anything, and probably would give us some post-traumatic stress. I agreed.

I really liked Mia. All day she had worn a giant purple sweater with a cat's face on it, complete with mixed media whiskers and a pink nose. Billie had gone ga-ga over the thing, and I was just happy see such a unique, colorful piece of clothing among the faded blue patterns of so many hospital gowns. If there was such a thing as psych ward style, Mia's cat-eye glasses, cat sweater, leggings, and slippers would have been on the cover of *Vogue*.

From the end of the hall, Angelique bounded out of the doorframe and motioned for us to hurry. "The sunset," she gushed. "It's amazing—you have to come see."

The dayroom didn't have the best view—we could not even see the skyline—but the sun's effect was magnificent. Many women were crowded around the windows, but even walking into the room, I could see the long rectangles of orange light on the dayroom floor. Peeking around shoulders, I saw the scene aglow; the sun lit up all of the roofs surrounding the hospital so that the city landscape below looked like an impressionist mosaic, with golds and scarlets and dark ambers and greens. The sky was a fierce, unapologetic yellow that faded to a pale blue, almost white, on one end and a bright golden orange toward the horizon. Just seeing all that light made me happier.

"Wow," Nina said.

"Isn't that something," someone agreed.

I leaned my head on Angelique's shoulder and just smiled, closing my eyes to capture the sunlight in my eyelids.

It was just a group of women, enjoying the sunset, huddled around two art-filled windows. I don't really know how to describe the sense of belonging that I felt in that moment. Maybe I was fresh off a high from my friends' visit, or maybe it was the fact that Venetia was now coming around with the snack cart and handing out bags of cheddar popcorn. I did not question it, I just enjoyed.

People started to trickle out or chase the sun as it curled past the horizon and lit up the clouds into even more brilliant colors. We were not allowed to step inside anyone else's rooms, so only the lucky eight or so with west-facing rooms were able to see the sun actually dip below the skyline. I was the very last one standing in front of the window and did not move until "Time for bed!" was called. Giving my head a little shake, I went back into my room to pull out Billie's turquoise marker and the legal pad Than had brought, and hid them under my pillow. After brushing my teeth and waiting for someone to check that was I in my room, I popped the cap off the marker as quietly as possible and started to pen my thoughts. I filled five pages without stopping, writing my favorite tidbits about my new friends, facts from The Night Of, bullet-points about my room, and as many details as I could remember about the past two days. I wrote lines about how being here was a challenge of faith, because being here meant trusting in a nameless system that we were never introduced formally to, a system that gave us butterfly coloring pages and packets of goldfish crackers as pacifiers.

Writing these scribbles meant I was forced into reflection, which is the last place I wanted to be at that hour, especially when the subject I was reflecting on was all this misery and anxiety and psychosis. After I had written all I could, I hid the notepad and marker in one of my brown paper bags and went to the nurse's station to ask for an Ambien. I swear to you, the nurse did not even ask a single question. She just scanned my patient wristband, logged the dosage into the computer, and handed me the plastic cup with the tiny pill inside. I sweetly said goodnight to the three nurses behind the glass, then returned to my room, slipped into the stiff covers, and waited for the medication to kick in.

For some reason, the children's book *Goodnight Moon* popped into my head at that moment, and I made a few psych ward verses in my head as it got foggier and foggier:

Goodnight beads
Goodnight barf
Goodnight penguin wearing a scarf
Goodnight nurses
Goodnight meds
Goodnight voices in Old Brenda's head
Goodnight slippers
Goodnight socks
And goodnight patients screaming, "Fuck off!"
Goodnight freedom
Goodnight fair
Goodnight crazies everywhere

III

Strategic Alliances

17

Maybe She's Born With It (Maybe It's Contraband)

I once had a substitute teacher who advised my class to always take offense if anyone said we looked tired. To the class of fifth graders, she explained that if a person said that, what they really meant was we looked awful.

That's what I thought of next morning when Billie matter-of-factly observed, "You look *exhausted*."

The Ambien had not worked as well as promised. I had woken up a handful of times in the middle of the night, prickling with sweat, so I was especially peeved when a nurse woke me up at 5:52 a.m. to take my yes-still-normal blood pressure. I know it was exactly that time because the counselor outside my door was berating someone, probably Gertrude or Billie, for walking the halls so early, saying, "Go back to bed! It's..." *Pause.* "...5:52 a.m.!"

But I had been too overheated to fall back asleep, so for an hour I just stared at the ceiling, listening for the sound of pacing footsteps outside my open door. It was impossible to get comfortable, and the bottom sheet was straight, not fitted, so all my tossing and turning shifted the linens around, and my sweaty skin kept sticking to the mat. Finally, I just sat up and stretched my back and shoulders. I rolled my head all the way around, making my neck crack like pond ice.

After getting up, I first ran into Nina. She was positively chipper. The meds they had given her yesterday had finally left her system, and it was great to see her back to the energetic woman I had met on Friday. I wished her a good morning and then passed to walk more swiftly. Billie caught up with me before I had even finished my first lap, the right half of her face spasming severely, as it did from time to time. I had barely greeted her before she delivered the brutal observation.

"Well, I *am* tired," I said, thinking that the bags under my eyes probably made me look like a cross between a panda and the loser in a fight. "And depressed."

"Yeah, well, what can I say," she shrugged. "This place is depressing."

"How'd you slee—" but she cut me off before I could finish and switched over to walking on my right side.

"Sorry," she said, pointing at her right ear. "Deaf, remember?"

"Right."

"Oh, and I want to give you a bracelet," she said, stopping and holding out her wrist. "You can have this one or this one. Not that one—that one was a gift."

"Wow, Billie, thanks."

I inspected her arm, recognizing the craft supplies immediately. Making up my mind, I chose the one with oddly shaped and severely mismatched beads, and Billie slipped it off her wrist and onto mine. I twisted it around a few times, admiring each unique bead, and knew I would wear it constantly or perhaps slip it onto my keychain once I left the hospital. It was a token—of friendship forged under ridiculous circumstances.

"Beautiful," she gushed, "just like you."

I rolled my eyes and gave her a one-armed hug, and we resumed our walk. On one of our laps, we passed Mia, still half-asleep and in her purple cat sweater, waiting to get her blood drawn.

"Did you know it's sixteen laps to a mile," Billie informed me.

"How the heck do you know that?" I said, incredulous at first. "Wait, I guess each of these squares is probably a foot."

"Exactly," Billie said. "And there's eighty on each length of the hall—I counted."

I did the math in my head. Eighty feet times four hallways per lap: 320 feet. 320 feet times sixteen laptops: five thousand feet and change. "Yeah—wow, that's really close."

"I walked like ten miles one day."

"Ten?" I said aghast.

"Well, there was nothing else to do! Before everyone came, people just stayed in their rooms! And that's just not healthy. So I had to move as much as possible—you know how I am."

I paused as we rounded the corner, finally adding, "That must have been really lonely."

"It was. But I at least I got my exercise!"

We neared Nina and Angelique walking toward us, both with their eyes peeled to the ground and scanning their gazes back and forth like metal detectors.

"Either of y'all see a skull bead?" Nina asked without looking up.

Angelique peered up, eyes red. "A red skull bead," she clarified. "It was on my bracelet and it's not here anymore. I must have lost it when—"

"We'll find it," Nina assured her before Angelique could start getting too worked up again.

"And we'll keep an eye out for it," I said. "Did it come from the bead bucket?"

"Yeah, and I just need to find it," Angelique said desperately. "I need to find it."

Nina turned back to us as Angelique continued searching the hallway floor. "She told me it reminds her of her boyfriend. It's gotta be here somewhere, unless someone took it."

"Maybe there's another one," I reasoned. "We can look today when Fiona comes."

Truthfully, I thought that was unlikely. The bucket held an impressive mixture of assorted store-bought craft bead styles. Over the years, as the bucket depleted, each new addition would have been poured onto the remains and now there had to be over fifty different styles all mixed together. For the unique beads, like the pink teddy bear I had seen the day before or the fat ribbed olive-colored bead on the bracelet gifted to me by Billie, there was little promise of finding a twin.

But that is not how you talk to someone who is stressed and fixated on a small problem to keep the tsunami of big problems at bay. So we would search all morning for that skull bead. And we would insist that even if it could not be found, there would be another.

I started rubbing the ribbed olive bead on my own wrist, just as a source of comfort. There was a pearly blue donut-shaped bead that felt good to spin too. As Billie and I continued walking, I kept my arms pretzeled in front of me, semi-consciously keeping a finger on my new favorite beads as we chatted and searched for Angelique's skull.

Billie was telling me that she took six showers yesterday, "...because of all this yelling! It makes me feel so icky and it makes me want to cry."

"Six showers," I marveled.

"This place is upsetting!" Billie said defensively.

"No, I hear you. I took an army shower from the sink."

"That how you like to take showers?"

"Not normally," I laughed. "My shower isn't getting hot water. Does yours?"

"Yeah, pretty hot. I mean, on and off, but it gets there."

"Think they'll let me use your shower?"

"Maybe, if you ask a nice one."

The thought of a hot shower was almost too much. Even with subpar water pressure, just having hot water running down my back, steam curling up all around me, would melt away some of the aches in my shoulders and perhaps ground my running thoughts, not to mention correct the greasiness of my hair.

"Just watch out for the silverfish," Billie added.

My two-second daydream halted.

Billie saw my look of revulsion. "Cold water or silverfish, you gotta decide."

"I choose no silverfish." I said resolutely.

"Good. They wouldn't have let you shower in my room anyway."

I smiled grimly and another wave of vertigo hit me. My hand flew to the wall to balance myself.

"Dizzy?"

"Yeah," I said. "Can we head to the dayroom? I can't walk anymore."

"Sure, hon. From your meds?"

"I guess. Who knows at this point."

Billie let out a sound of sympathy, and we lumbered to the dayroom. One of the staff was leaving with a wide broom, having just finished sweeping. She gave us no greeting, unless you count her clucking her tongue as we crossed her path to get to the big table.

"Excuse you," said Billie.

I looked around for the newspaper, but it either was not there or had already been snatched up by an earlier bird.

Billie bent down to inspect the floor underneath the table. "Disgusting," she remarked. "She didn't even sweep under here!"

I squatted down next to her and indeed, there were paper scraps, crumbs, and beads in high concentration.

"Maybe Angelique's bead is down here," I mused. I scanned the linoleum tiles and picked up at least ten beads, cupping each in my palm to inspect more closely before pouring them into a spare Syrofoam cup. No red skulls.

"I bet they don't even clean the tables in here," Billie criticized. She dragged a finger across the tabletop. "And look, there's still tons of shit on this floor! Did they even *try* to clean this room?"

"Why would they? Visitors go to Dayroom B. No one ever sees this one."

"That has to violate some health code or something."

"Don't think they're too worried."

Angelique and Nina wandered in, Angelique still searching the floors and looking crestfallen. Nina at least had more pep in her step. She was grinning at us, still wearing her crown of beads, red hair braided and resting on her shoulder.

"I decided I'm not going to take my pill today," she told us.

"It made me feel awful yesterday."

I shot her two thumbs up. "Hell yeah."

Normally, I am all for adhering to a medication regimen, wholly trusting that whatever is prescribed is for the best. But having seen the haphazardness of new med prescriptions around here, and how pills seemed to just be chosen with about as much thought as orders at a fast food restaurant, I had little faith in Nina's doctor. This was especially true after comparing Nina's behavior yesterday to her behavior on Friday.

"They won't just let you *not* take it," Angelique said.

Nina pretended not to hear her and instead gazed happily at the sun shining through the window.

When the silver food cart finally arrived, I was already sweaty, hungry, and uncomfortable. On the bright side, my tray had everything I had ordered: Frosted Flakes and milk; a cup of unripe cantaloupe and soft grapes; a blueberry muffin, sausage patty, and a scoop of eggs; and coffee, hot chocolate, *and* tea. By hospital accounts, a full Sunday brunch buffet. I tucked the teabag and hot chocolate packet into the waistband of my pants and then offered up my eggs and sausage to the table, looking to Big Brenda first. Then I poured milk into my cereal bowl and spooned my first bite of Frosted Flakes in years. Sweet and crunchy, just like I remembered.

While we were all eating and swapping plates, Nurse Avery came in with the tray of meds and water cups. The meds were distributed, including Nina's, and the nurse eyed each patient as we tossed back the little plastic cup into our mouths. On the whole, I was starting to prefer this new Cymbalta to my old sertraline; these new capsules were not giving me any heartburn, whereas the sertraline tablets had me in the habit of always carrying Tums.

I was halfway through my muffin before I noticed Nina grinning at me.

"It's in my milk!" she mouthed, pointing at her open carton and then underneath her tongue.

I raised a fist in victory.

Angelique, the crafty genius, figured out that by mixing Vaseline and oil pastels swiped from the craft cart, you can make psych ward-quality makeup, so by mid-morning she had bright red puckering lips, and Nina had dark brown eyebrows again. No staff members had come to run a group therapy session, so we asked a counselor to drag out the bead bucket. Then the newspaper delivery person finally arrived and dropped the Sunday paper onto the side table with a heavy thud. Little Brenda divvied it up. She handed the crossword to me, kept the adverts for herself, and then distributed the comics evenly between Mary and Big Brenda. Delilah pulled her reading glasses out of her pocket and flipped to the front page of the business section like a Suburban father straight from the fifties.

Nina switched chairs in order to sit next to me and read off everyone's horoscopes from the column beside my crossword clues.

"What's it say for Aquarius?" Billie called out.

Nina dragged her finger down the line and cleared her throat. "Says a lover from the past is going to surprise you today."

"Hey, maybe that means my ex-husband found a way to spring me out of here!" Billie deduced.

"Good, you've been here too long," I said. "What about for Libra?"

"Oh, I'm a Libra too! It says..." and Nina mumbled under her breath before giving us her interpretation. "It says it's a good day to 'take a well-deserved rest'?"

"Oh God!" Billie exclaimed. "That's every day in here. Did some asshole write those just to fuck with us?"

"I doubt the doctors have access to the newspaper publishers," I told her.

She raised her eyebrows at me meaningfully and opened her mouth, but before she could start spouting conspiracies and disrupting the morning serenity, I interrupted.

"Hey, you wanted me to paint you something, right? For your room? Why don't you pick out a page and I can paint it if Fiona comes today with the watercolors."

Billie considered it and then walked to the stack of coloring sheets. She chose a detailed idyll of a cottage surrounded by a wreath of ivy and flowers, but then moved on to reading off the group therapy schedule posted on the back wall.

"Did we have a Discharge Planning Group yesterday? No we did not. What about current events? Don't think so! And a movie? Ha!"

Maybe Billie should have been born a Libra.

One of the newest patients, a grumpy Black woman with two-inch nails, finally yelled at Billie, "Shut up! No one cares!" which only made Billie shout back, "That's fine! I'm advocating for all of us. I don't care if you appreciate it or not!"

"Why don't you try to get us someone who can run group?" Nina suggested diplomatically.

"Yeah," agreed Little Brenda. "It's Sunday. Shouldn't we have Spiritual Group?"

"Good i-de-a," Billie replied, emphasizing each syllable. "I'll go see if I can find the chaplain."

As Billie exited stage right, Mia came in, said hello, grabbed a discarded magazine and a few glossy pages from the plucked over newspaper, and left again. I started pulling all colors and hues of donut-shaped beads out of the bucket, getting to over two dozen before a single shade repeated. Then Fiona came in, the craft cart in tow, before mentioning she was due on another floor.

"I brought you more beads though," Fiona announced, then pausing as if for applause. "Since you girls love them so much!"

Angelique made a beeline for the new bucket, tore off the plastic, and started sifting through for the twin of her beloved skull. Fiona backed out of the room, wide hips swaying, transitioning to an awkward shuffling trot after she rounded the corner.

"Is there any more string?" Angelique inquired, as I stood to grab a tray of watercolors.

I only saw two-inch scraps of that red plasticky string. "Think we used it all up yesterday," I reported.

"Fiona, can you get us more?"

"She's already gone. Had to go to Fourteen."

"Quick when she wants to be, isn't she?" Billie said, already returning from wherever she had been and whomever she had been drilling.

"Find a chaplain?" asked Little Brenda.

"Yeah, he's signing in."

Billie came over to me, where I had started a wash of green on the outer ivy of her idyll. She gasped in delight, even though there was nothing to be delighted at yet, and hugged my shoulders. I added as many colors to the picture as I could, thinking about how the sun would catch each one and brighten up Billie's dreary hospital room. Two kinds of blue on the birds. Four shades of red and pink on the flowers. Orange and ochre and the cleanest yellow I could manage from this overmixed paint tray. Polka dots of purple. Stripes of lime green. Indigo details on the leaves.

It did not take very long to finish, and I was just presenting it to Billie when the Chaplain knocked on the open door. But like Fiona, he could not stay for very long. He gave us an apology as a greeting and asked who wanted to start with a prayer. I grabbed the newspaper crossword and headed back to my room for a different kind of spiritual ceremony.

When I was alone in my room, I propped myself up against the wall and gazed at a blank page of the legal pad. Yellow paper, green lines. With Billie's marker, I scribbled a deluge of unfiltered thoughts. The more I wrote, the tighter my chest felt. I rubbed the comforting olive bead on my wrist.

I did not want to be here anymore. It was not the routine that was stifling—I even wished there was more of one, with group therapy that I could count on and that actually served a purpose. Without a doubt, it was the feeling that this place was keeping me stalled. I was here, forcibly being kept on pause, while the world sped ahead without me. I was not making any sort of progress in these white walls, in this square ward with screaming patients. I still had not even seen a proper psychiatric doctor.

I had come to the hospital feeling like I was dying, and instead of patching me up, this place had just put me on ice.

If it had been a normal Sunday, I would be running errands today. I might have had brunch with Than and Kevin and then caught a movie at the Logan Theater. I would be enjoying this good weather and wearing a dress and perhaps making plans to see a concert or grill on someone's rooftop. Instead, I was trapped in a hospital and inside my own mind.

Patty had been discharged last night, leaving just before snack time. I had not seen her leave, I had just heard through the rumor mill that she was gone. Apparently, they give you a bus ticket and an exit survey, and then just send you back into the big bad world. Patients were coming in and leaving all the time and still, but I had zero information about my own discharge plan. What if I was a clerical error, and I was due to leave today but someone had just forgotten to tell me? It seemed unlikely but, given the unorganized state of everything around here, also possible.

Deciding I would get some information for myself, I marched purposefully over to Yulia, who sat stationed at the counselor's desk in front of the nurse's station.

"Hi," I said tersely.

She looked up at me, about to smile, and then saw the look on my face. "Can I help with something?"

"Yes. Yes. I want to know when I can be discharged."

"I'm not sure. Only a doctor or a nurse practitioner can discharge you."

"Any idea when I can see one of those?" I asked, not breaking eye contact. I felt slightly bad for being so abrasive with Yulia because she was one of the nice ones. She just had the misfortune of being on guard while I was in search of answers.

"Maybe ask the nurses?" She offered, indicating the three women behind the windows of the nurse's station. "They might know."

So I knocked on the glass, growing frustrated when none of them immediately turned around or rushed to meet me at the door. Finally, a nurse named Joanne turned away from the computer where she was entering notes and saw me on the other side of the window.

"Hello, what's up?" Joanne said from the door. She was petite, had long dark brown hair, and reminded me of someone I went to high school with. "Need anything?"

"*How do you know my name!*"

Greta's raised voice leaked out of the day room. Joanne closed her eyes in silent commiseration as one of her peers tried to get Greta to take her late-morning meds.

I ignored the distraction and cleared my throat. "Do you know when a doctor or a nurse practitioner will be in? I'm trying to find out when I can be discharged."

"Dr. Moran should be here this afternoon." Joanne answered, before Greta's continued protest prompted her to shout over her shoulder, "Need help in there?"

Unsatisfied, I probed further. "Like two o'clock?"

"Probably," Joanne said, then adding, "I think they'll probably let you leave soon. You go to group, take your meds, don't cause any trouble. They might even let you leave tomorrow."

My heart skipped. "Cool, thanks," I said, starting to walk away. Then I turned around again and mouthed a more sincere, "Thank you," which I am not sure she saw as she ran toward the sound of Greta shouting, "I can't take that!"

Tomorrow! That was the answer I had been hoping for; even though I had not seen a psychiatrist since being here, Joanne said this was possible. I could be less than twenty-four hours away from fresh air, the best of Chicago's restaurants, and sleeping in my own bed. Maybe I could even talk this Dr. Moran into letting Than take me home tonight!

Because three days was a lifetime in here. On the outside, three days pass by in a blink. Three days in the real world is just over half a workweek, three times punching in, three times punching out. You could stay in bed for an entire three days,

147

only getting up to use the bathroom and eat granola bars, and no one would even bat an eye.

I am speaking from experience here. My job as a consultant had me traveling out of O'Hare Mondays at dawn and returning Thursday evenings. Then, some Fridays, I chose not to go into the office, preferring to dial into meetings from my bed and then staying there watching Netflix until it was time to repack my suitcase Sunday night. Sometimes that is all I have the energy for, and with no boyfriend, two roommates with their own busy schedules, and a bed on the far side of the apartment, there might be no external force all weekend to coax me out of my room.

Now that kind of weekend nearly describes the weekend I was currently having—a boring, sedentary one where all I do is mope—but there are some very important distinctions, and I do not think you need me to spell them out for you. You have been with me this far.

What I am trying to explain is that three days is nothing. Except in here. I needed to get the hell out, or at least know where the finish line was, so I could keep it in my sights.

I went to go find Mia to tell her that a doctor was coming soon. She was not in either dayroom still, so I started poking my head into the rooms on the north wall. I found her sitting cross-legged on her bed, still in her purple cat sweater and cat-eye glasses, surrounded by ripped magazine pages.

I tapped on her own door. "Hi."

"What's up?"

"One of the nurses told me Dr. Moran's coming in later, so we'll be able to find out about getting discharged."

"About fucking time!"

I stood awkwardly in her doorway, watching her place

colorful magazine segments around a piece of paper.

"What are you making?" I asked tentatively.

"It's a collage," she said, holding it up. "I've been using Vaseline instead of glue. And ripping the paper, since there's no scissors."

I considered it. Mia had and snatched a number of faces, including a smoky-eyed Natalie Portman, out of their glossy settings and Picasso'd them onto the blank page. The words "MENTAL BREAK" sat across the top.

"Nice," I said.

"I think it accurately captures the insanity of what I'm feeling in here."

"Show me when it's finished?" Mia nodded and I backed out of her door frame before the counselor on duty could tell me not to stick my nose in other people's rooms.

There was still plenty of time before lunch, but there was nothing I wanted to do. I was at a standstill with my crosswords and, with such frequent hallway interruptions, none of Than's books I had cracked were keeping my attention. I even tried playing tic-tac-toe with some of the Kittens, figuring it would be like playing with a five-year-old, but Mary and Francine both got along fine without me and even seemed to prefer a loss to a draw. They would both cheer for each other, no matter who won, while I just could not bring myself to pretend to care. I considered starting a game of hangman on the whiteboard with Angelique and Nina, but the thought of a counselor walking in and seeing a scribbled hangman's rig made me smile wryly and pass on the idea.

I guess I could shower. Basic hygiene, never a bad idea. And since boredom felt like drowning anyway, I might as well add some water.

18

Getting Clean

Back in high school, I would take a full course load of AP classes, followed by anywhere from two to three clubs after school and then around six hours of homework a night, so I used showers as my daily retreat. I think most people might do that, but I also think I took it too far. If I did not take my 7:00 p.m. shower, I would be panicking by 7:15 p.m.

It was my chance to take a break from the stress, to let the soap and steam melt it away and allow me to pretend that there were not five more hours of assignments and reading to tackle as soon as I towel-dried my hair. I cried so much in high school—and since this was before I knew much about mental illness, how common it is, and how I might be affected by it, these tears were intensely isolating. The confines of the shower made my misery private and even more dramatic—just how I thought it should be.

But right now, I was not interested in amplifying the misery of my feelings. I just wanted everything to fast forward.

Without stripping off my clothes, I turned the handle on my shower and prayed for the water to heat up. By some miracle, it reached an acceptable lukewarm temperature, and I undressed, closed the bathroom curtain, and grabbed the combination shampoo-conditioner and bar of soap faster than Big Brenda ate last night's dinner roll.

Goosebumps shot up on my calves and arms, but I rubbed them down and splashed water on as much of my body as possible. Knowing even the lukewarm water temperature might not last long, I rubbed soap into my hair with vigor and then dragged the bar of soap across all my limbs and stomach. I rinsed off slowly. It still smelled like a public swimming pool shower, and the water temperature was starting to chill, but if I closed my eyes and breathed in the slight smell of chlorine, I could imagine that I had just finished swimming laps in a pool while on vacation. Or that I had just had a sun-filled afternoon on the water slide in the St. Louis Park water park. Or that I had been practicing how long I could hold my breath in the gigantic fifteen-foot-deep pool at the Williston Athletic Club, or the neighbor's pool, or the pool at FOSS Swim School where I first took lessons. If I just focused on the water stream dripping down my back, I did not feel as trapped.

When I finished showering, I wrapped the tiny towel around my midriff and used one of my cleaner tees to wring out my hair. I did not bother attempting to brush it, just twisted it up into a messy knot held together by the one hair tie I had come in with. That hair tie was on its last legs. The elastic had broken and was being held together by the black string encasing it. I swear, if that thing finally snapped, I would too.

There was still some time before lunch, which I tried to kill with a half-hearted nap and another attempt at getting into a new book. It was exhausting, trying to fill the time. Doing nothing was hard.

There was a new face at our table when I finally sat down with my tray at lunch. Nina introduced her to all of us as Jennifer and told us how she had come in the night before after being relocated from a rehab center that would not take her insurance.

"My boyfriend and I are gonna get clean," she shared with us. She told us she had been smoking dope for half her life, that it was time to stop, and that she hoped she could. "But this isn't really the place to do it, huh? No way this place'll give me methadone."

"They've got the patch," Big Brenda told her.

"Yeah, and the gum," Nina said from Jennifer's immediate left. Sitting next to each other, Jennifer looked like Nina's younger sister. She had her dark red hair tied back in a messy braid too, and although she had fewer wrinkles and was slimmer, she had the same skin and posture. They even talked similarly.

"So this is lunch?" Jennifer asked me, nodding at her tray. "Why don't I have what you have?"

"It's your first day," I responded, "so you got the standard tray. Tomorrow you'll get a menu and can customize what you want."

"How's the coffee?"

"It's decaf. But tomorrow morning, order the hot chocolate and save the packets. You can get hot water out of your bathroom faucet."

"I don't want to eat any of this," Jennifer said dejectedly. "Anyone want it?"

"Me," Big Brenda said, reaching across two people for Jennifer's dried out french fries.

"Can I have your fruit?" Billie asked.

"Go ahead. I got zero appetite. Is this how lunch always is?"

I passed on all my veteran's knowledge, including how the fruit cup was usually just unripe melon, and you would be lucky if they got half of your order right. I immediately liked Jennifer, and I wanted her to like me. She was down-to-earth, seemed confident, and exuded a type of effortless cool that I would not have expected to find in someone who had been shoved into a psych ward for trying to get clean.

Lunch was particularly unappetizing that day, so most of us had pushed our trays away before long. I had eaten part of the roll and nibbled on the sad-looking deli sandwich. Mia had finally been given a meal that passed as vegetarian, but the pile of cottage cheese on her plate kept making me think of Delilah's vomit from before, and I was concentrating on controlling my gag reflex. Billie was chattering away about something or other, and Nina and Angelique were back to digging through the beads.

"So what's it like in here?" Jennifer was asking. After getting only weak shrugs and contorted faces from around the table, she followed up with, "Then what's there to do?"

"Drawing." That was Angelique.

"Napping." That was Mia.

"Hang out." Nina.

"Walk around." Billie.

Jennifer made a different face for each suggestion. "Is there anything to read?"

"I've got some books," I offered. "Want to pick one out?"

Jennifer agreed and stood up with me. Her hair swished across her shoulders as she followed me back to my room, and I could feel my heart beating harder for some reason. As she thumbed through the titles I had lined up on my storage shelf, I leaned against the wall and watched her from over my glasses. She had a beautifully unique face and, as she read the back of every book carefully, she chewed her lip as her steely eyes moved down the cover.

I had strategically closed my door as much as possible behind us. This was as much privacy as I could give us.

"Do you know why I wanted you to come in here?" I said as calmly as I could.

She met my gaze and smiled slightly when she saw my intent expression. "Why's that?" she whispered.

I moved closer to her and, resting my hands on either side of her face, breathed, "I just wanted to get you alone."

Then I leaned in and took her mouth in mine.

19

Who Ya Gonna Call?

Kidding!

There are no psych ward lesbian lovers in this story. Sorry if you got excited there—I just needed a laugh.

In reality, I brought my books out to her in the hallway—because we are not allowed in each other's rooms, remember? She glanced at my collection and decided on *A Clockwork Orange,* and we made our way back down the hall.

"Thanks, I appreciate it," Jennifer said, already cracking the book open.

"No problem. If you don't like that one, just come back and swap it out."

"Cool. I don't know how everybody survives in here without stuff to do."

"Well, if you could call it surviving," I joked. "I've been here since Thursday night and I think my IQ's dropped ten points."

"Shit," she said. "Do you know where I can get some of that nicotine gum they were talking about?"

"Probably the nurse's station." I pointed her down the hall and told her I would meet her back in Dayroom A. "It's where the cool kids sit."

Billie had convinced one of the counselors to let us run our own bingo game, and they were distributing bingo chips and boards when I got back. Somehow Billie had even managed to squirrel away so many snacks that her black-market bingo had prizes.

Francine, Mary, Big Brenda, Little Brenda, Angelique, and some of the new patients were all sitting placidly inside. Styrofoam cups full of colorful bingo chips were placed evenly around the center table, with Billie at the head, the crank of the bingo cage ready in her hand.

"Everyone that wants to play, get ready!" Billie called. She turned to me and asked, "You in?"

But at that moment, I realized how socially worn out I was. "I think I'm just going to lie down," I said. I immediately saw her face fall and felt bad as I turned away. But my patience was wearing thin, and I needed to rest up before meeting with Dr. Moran. It was important that I made a good impression. I did not like disappointing Billie by not joining her spontaneous bingo game, but my goal was to get out, not play games. And anyway, the room smelled like farts again.

"You leaving?" Jennifer asked as she passed me by the door.

"Yeah. Tired."

"Oh, okay," she said, smacking her Nicorette. "Catch you later."

Back in my room, I sat dejectedly on the side of my bed. Twenty seconds ago, all I wanted was to be alone, and now all I wanted was to be with other people. What the hell was that about?

I grabbed *Winter's Bone* off my shelf and turned to where I had left off. The protagonist, Ree Dolly, was tough. She took no shit, even when shit was all she had. I generally make a point to never compare tough situations because there is nothing to be gained from playing Who Has It Worse, but I was finding some comfort in reading about a character who had it bad. Misery loves company and all that.

My mind wandered to consider who I would be calling during phone hours that evening. Probably just Than again. I toyed around with the idea of calling my other roommate, but I did not want to interrupt him while he was enjoying a short vacation with his girlfriend. I could call my dad, but it would feel like an emotional expense to shatter his illusion of The Competent Daughter, and I could not handle that at the moment. Maybe my mom—but then I would have to explain why I was calling from an unrecognized number, and when she found out, she would either fly down to smother me with compensatory motherhood or reframe the situation until it was unrecognizable. Than's mom, possibly; Jen is sharp, clever, action-oriented. Liberal in both her politics and her amount of maternal affection. I could call her, no questions asked. But the thought of doing that felt hard too.

I was suddenly craving small talk, even though it would tire me out after ten minutes. And if I was honest with myself, I was also craving another person's touch, to be held and cared for by someone who loved me romantically and unconditionally. I missed the feeling of being in love, even if I had never felt it perfectly before.

I thought about the ex who had just gotten engaged. He had initially gone from being just a high school distraction to being a close friend. Then in college, we had sprinkled in some benefits, talked through his betrayals, and then dated erroneously, all the while caring profoundly for one another.

But now, he was engaged and off-limits to me. He had found a different happiness, and I was not going to call him for fifteen minutes of catching up and comfort if it meant there was a risk of upsetting his newfound balance. I knew he might be tempted to deny that his ex-girlfriend was calling him out of the blue in order to protect his fiancée's feelings.

A year ago, I Skyped him once when I was feeling low. That is how I met his fiancée for the first time—he had answered the call while in bed with her, and she was nuzzled up against him, with only her eyes peeking out from under their shared blanket. It was a fresh start for him, free from the dysfunction that had riddled our immature relationship. After that, I stopped reaching out, partly because I did not want to get in the way but also because it hurt too much to see him that happy. The if-only-we-had-waited game was too painful. But of all the relationships, both long and short, he had always been the one I wanted to run to and fight for.

I thought about Jack, the guy who I had slept with for months, who had become a close friend, and who I had all intentions of dating until he finally revealed to me that he did not want to be in a relationship at his age. My girlfriends had comforted me by saying he was just immature and that maturity was So Important, but I appreciated that he was at least mature enough to recognize what he did not want, even if I could not really understand the reasons why. We were still close, still figuring out how to coexist in our shared neighborhood in Chicago. Alone in this psych ward room, with the words of *Winter's Bone* blurring before my eyes, I thought about him and wished he was sitting at the edge of this bed, stroking my hair like he used to do after a long day.

Maybe I could call him. But I did not know his number by

heart, and Than would not have it either, so with my phone dead and locked in the contraband closet, Jack could have been as far as Thailand, and it would not have made a difference.

I thought back to Jennifer's question from lunch, "What's it like here?" I was sure that once I got out, people would ask me that same question. *What was it like inside the psych ward? Did they administer electro-shock therapy? Did they hide the pills in pudding? Did they strap you to the beds?*

If my life outside had been semi-miserable comfort, then this was semi-comfortable misery. We were fed three times a day and we had our own toilets, and I would certainly qualify that as comfortable enough, especially since this was clearly an under-resourced hospital system (or perhaps it *was* adequately-resourced, and funds were just never properly diverted to the adult behavioral floors). But there was also no denying that this was a place of misery. A ward of hopelessness to quarantine the dejected and degenerate from polite society. A pen for fucked up people.

I keep a notebook of tidbits and advice I receive or think up, and often I forget to attribute them. So I cannot remember if this one came from me, someone else, or some post on Pinterest, but one of my nuggets is this: Don't let yourself feel miserable just so others can feel comfortable.

There were plenty of times when I have felt disinclined to reach out for help, too afraid to alter a status quo or upset the peace. Like, say I am at a party, and one hour in, all the stimulation—pounding bass, gyrating bodies, small talk—starts to trigger a panic attack. So I take refuge in the nearest bathroom, splash some water on my face, try to give myself a pep talk in the mirror and diffuse the pressure in my chest. Sometimes this works, but sometimes this just dissolves into me hogging up the bathroom and trying to cry silently so as not to disturb the festivities outside.

Crying on a toilet lid or on the edge of a tub in a stranger's bathroom while a crowd parties just on the other side of the door always feels like rock bottom. And from that perch, there are three options: stay inside to occupy the bathroom indefinitely and be miserable, swap my tears for a peppy mask and return to the party only to be miserable, or go find my friends who I came to the party with and be a lot less miserable. Taking the third option is not easy, because it comes with the knowledge that I am putting my friends in an uncomfortable spot by asking them to sacrifice their night of revelry in exchange for a much less fun one of Making Sure Cosette Is Okay. So sometimes I take the second option and pull an Irish exit shortly thereafter. But I try to take Option Three. Good friends encourage you to take Option Three and I have good friends.

Don't let yourself feel miserable just so others can feel comfortable. Good friends will not find helping you to be *un*comfortable anyway.

Oh, and another piece of advice from my little notebook: Find good friends and put everything you have got into those friendships. Trust me, it is a lifesaver.

20

Falling On Deaf Ears

At 2:15 p.m., an orderly knocked on my door to tell me I was supposed to talk to Dr. Moran.

"He's already here?" I asked, irritated that no one had told me, but the orderly was already onto the next door.

I bolted upright and ran to the bathroom to inspect myself. Hair was tangled, so I tried to brush. Eyes were bleary, so I put a wet washcloth over them. Outfit was absurd, but I had no clothing that could help that, so nothing to be done there.

By the time I walked up to the tiny office room, there was already a line of patients wrapping around the corner. Mia was just coming out by the time I took my place at the back of the line, and I motioned for her to come over. Her face was deadpan and eyes drooping, so I could not get any sort of read on her.

"What did he say?" I pestered intently. "How soon can you get out?"

"Tuesday morning. I told him that I'm going to that intensive in-patient place I was telling you about, so he had to let me."

"That's great! That's great, right?"

"Yeah, it's whatever."

"Were you hoping for sooner?" I asked.

"Eh. That's about what I figured. I'm just so sick of this place."

"You and me both," I said quietly.

Mia trudged away with another word, leaving me to crane my neck to count the number of heads in front of me. Five, including Francine and Big Brenda.

The next woman to exit was the Black woman who had arrived at the same time as Jennifer. Earlier, I had learned her name was Deondra when I overheard one of the nurses call her a "fighter" and now, she came out of the tiny office, fists waving in the air. She addressed us, ranting, "Bitches, don't let those motherfuckers talk to you like that, like they're the fucking kings of the universe. They don't know nothin'! Stupid ass motherfuckers need to let me the fuck *out*!"

Everyone in line averted eye contact, which only made her yell louder. Francine whimpered and then rolled her wheelchair into the office. Big Brenda looked like she was willing to get in a fight, but before she could start yelling back at the woman, one of the orderlies yelled in our direction and waved a syringe in the air threateningly.

Francine's consultation went much more peacefully, and she rolled out with a demure smile on her face. Big Brenda's went quickly, and she mouthed, "Tomorrow!" at me on her way out. My stomach fluttered. I could not remember how many days Big Brenda had said she had been there before I arrived, but here was proof that this Dr. Moran was at least letting people out.

When I was finally at the front of the line, I realized how

anxious I was. My hands were sweating profusely, and my heart was going at probably 120 beats per minute even though I was standing still. Should I go in and shake his hand? Would that demonstrate competence and prove that I was fit to engage with the real world? I had plenty of experience making good impressions for teachers and clients. Did the same concepts apply to psychiatrists?

When the woman who had been ahead of me in line exited, I took a deep breath and turned to enter the room. But before I could get both feet across the threshold, Joanne, the nurse with long brown hair and tired eyes, said, "Just a moment. We'll call you in we're ready," and shut the door.

What the hell? They had not shut the door before any of the other patients went in. Why did they need special time to prepare for me?

I had seen just a glimpse of the room inside, and it truly was tiny. A tall person probably could have reached their arms out and touched both walls, but somehow they had crammed in a full-size desk, a file cabinet, and two oversized office chairs with a plastic chair for the patient. I had only seen Dr. Moran for a split-second, and my first impression was that he looked like one of the monsters from that children's book, *Where the Wild Things Are.* His skin was purplish-grey and heavily peppered with moles. He had a large nose, drooping eyes that reminded me of a basset hound, and thick black hair streaked with grey that grew out of a massive forehead. He had literal jowls.

My heart beat even faster, but it was hardly a full minute before Joanne opened the door again. "Sorry about that. Just had to finish up some notes. Come on in."

Joanne took the seat next to the doctor, holding a clipboard and sitting with her back straight. Dr. Moran peered at the slip of paper Joanne had pushed in front of him and read aloud, "1525...Hay-jen."

I cringed internally at the awkward mispronunciation of my name but smiled and made no correction. "Hi. That's me."

"And how are you doing?" he asked, not looking up from the desk. He had a deep but weak, monotonous voice that made my overly cheerful voice sound even more over-the-top.

"I'm doing better." I said, serving up the answer I thought was best.

Dr. Moran looked at Joanne. "She said she's doing fine," Joanne repeated loudly. She shot me an apologetic look, adding, "He doesn't hear so well."

"How is the..." he squinted his eyes at the page, "Cymbalta? Thirty milligrams."

"Um, it's fine," I said, talking a little louder. "Doesn't feel all that different right now. But I'm definitely feeling withdrawal symptoms from my old medication, sertraline. I was hoping that I could taper off of it—"

"Sertraline?" Dr. Moran asked Joanne, interrupting me mid-sentence.

"Yes, that's what she used to take! She's saying she feels *with-draw-al* symptoms!"

Dr. Moran looked back at his page. "Hm." A long silence. Then he added, "How do you feel?"

"About what?" I said, still using my forcefully cheery tone. "Like, depression-wise?"

"Yes. Depression."

"I'm okay. I'm dizzy and sweaty and a little nauseous, but I think that's just from switching meds so quickly like that. Mostly I'm pretty anxious still, but it's hard not to be in here with all the screaming and stuff. I'm not sleeping that well, either."

I did not know what else to say. Under the desk, my legs were bouncing nervously, and I gripped my thumbs in my lap. Based on the doctor's monotonous tone, lack of eye contact, and the fact that he could *barely hear a word I said*, I did not feel like this consultation was going well.

"Let's increase her dosage to sixty milligrams." Dr. Moran said to Joanne, who wrote the number down on her clipboard.

"When do you think I can get out?" I asked boldly. "Because I was thinking, since I've been going to all the grou—"

"It will be good for you to stay until at least Wednesday."

Wednesday. My heart sank, and tears instantly welled up in my eyes, an annoying reaction to disappointment. "Not Tuesday?"

"Wednesday, I think. We will increase your meds, and give them time to work."

"But I'm feeling better now. And I'm self-admitted. Not suicidal."

"Wednesday, at the earliest."

"I really think it would be better for me if—"

"She's been going to all the groups and she has been a very good patient," Joanne interjected.

But Dr. Moran was already writing his decision down with pen and reciting it out loud. "You were admitted on Thursday at midnight, and five days for this type of admittance is typical."

I could feel the tears brimming, and any minute they would spill over my eyelashes. Wednesday was a lifetime away. It meant that I was not even halfway through my stay. This guy knew me by my room number better than by my name and had talked to me for less than five minutes, but somehow he had the authority to serve me this sentence without even a second's further consideration. And how was I supposed to be able to explain anything, communicate anything, when the man *could not even fucking hear?*

I had tuned out the second half of his bumbling and finally, just as the tears were about to spill, I interrupted him and stood up. Turning to Joanne, I said loudly, "Can I go? He's not telling me anything of value to my health."

She nodded sympathetically, and I turned on my heel and walked out of the teeny closet, hoping that the useless doctor felt as insulted and disrespected by my exit as I had by his patient care.

I was fuming. And crying. I walked straight past the nurses and counselors at the nurse's station and made a beeline for my room, letting out the first ugly sob just as I turned the corner.

It took all the self-control I had in me not to slam the door once I arrived in 1525. This was not *my* room, I thought to myself, cursing the numbers stamped on the orange plastic placard. This was a temporary inhabitancy. And I was not a number. I did not belong here, in this clinical room, with the bed that could not even touch the walls and the bathroom that was not allowed a door. I paced around, fists clenched at my side, knowing full well that there was no furniture I could physically toss, and my window artwork would not even tear down satisfyingly since it was stuck up with goopy Vaseline. There was nothing to wreck, nothing to ruin, and I so wanted to tear at my own arms and legs and torso. I wanted to draw blood, even if it was my own.

My full-on internal meltdown had no outlet in which to

explode, so I fell face-first onto the thin mattress, hitting my forehead on the metal platform underneath. I sobbed heavily into the pillow, not caring that the sound would barely be muted. Fuck that Dr. Moran. What a fucking Moranster.

Do you remember those old public service ads that showed an egg in a frying pan and went, "This is your brain on drugs. Any questions?" Well, allow me to demonstrate my brain on anxiety:

...If I stayed here for too long, my life would unravel at the seams. I would lose all momentum on my project at work. I would lose the relationships with clients I had worked so hard to establish. Once everyone heard about this, no one would want to work with me ever again. I would probably be fired for being a liability. Or, maybe even worse, I would be "encouraged to pursue other opportunities" that were less demanding and more appropriate for my fragile mental state.

...My friends would try to be supportive. We would go to brunch and they would ask me how my search for a new job was going. They would ask, gazes averted, about how I had been feeling, and then their sighs of relief would give them away that yes, of course, they were only asking to be polite. Eventually, they would stop inviting me out for fear of setting me off. Or perhaps first they would all leave Chicago, forget about me, and I would never see them again. I would just be a sad, lonely Chicagoan who never strayed outside of her rented apartment except to bring in the Instacart grocery delivery.

Or maybe I would never even be allowed to leave the hospital. Maybe the doctors would never let me leave, and I would wallow away, slowly covering up the window with childish pictures until I could no longer see the rectangular houses below. Meanwhile, the cost of keeping me in this place would drain my bank account. Insurance would demand payment, and I would drown in debt faster than I would drown in sorrow. Then the hospital would *kick* me out, and I would join the five-thousand homeless people in Chicago. I would huddle under the overpass near the Belmont CTA Station and ask for mercy from the frigid winter wind.

Or maybe my family would feel pressured to foot the bill. My younger siblings would have to travel across two state lines to visit their invalid sister. Their eyes would be as round as the trampoline we played on, and they wouldn't understand how the sister that baked them Rice Krispie Treats could be the same person with greasy hair and square socks that they saw now. My mother would wail at the heavens, angry at how this could happen to her daughter, and my father and stepmom would wonder how they missed the signs. The neighbors would try to talk., but they would not know what to say.

I would miss my ten year high school reunion, and everyone would whisper about how the once-upon-a-time National Merit Scholar who had delivered their graduation speech was now rotting away behind a locked door. My college professors would shake their heads with pity and wonder how, after graduating Summa Cum Laude with three majors, I could have strayed so far from success. They would recall to themselves, "I guess she did always seem a little high strung."

Within a month, I would become unrecognizable. I would stop showering. I would never leave my room. I would forget what fresh air tasted like, and eventually be choked by the artificial and antiseptic AC being pumped in through the vents. If I stayed any longer, everything would be lost. Life would be over. There was no doubt in my restless, rattled mind.

Any questions?

21

Everybody Cries

My thoughts had run a marathon, but I had only been sprawled out on my mat for around five minutes. But after I had mentally played out every disaster scenario, the calm that comes too quickly fell upon me. Survival demands action, and I was now in survival mode. The best way to survive is to be reasonable, and that meant considering the facts. The Moranster may have been a shitty doctor, but he had to be basing his shitty decisions on something—some policy or written advisory, perhaps. At least, that is what reason figured.

The counselor Mohammed was on duty across the hall from my door, and I was still tear-stricken and hiccupping when I approached him.

"Bad news," he said, matter-of-factly.

I sighed heavily. "But he wouldn't tell me *why*. How am I supposed to get out sooner if he doesn't tell me that?"

Mohammed searched my face and then turned to his computer screen. He clicked and scrolled a bit, then turned back to me. "It's because of your chart."

I snapped upright. "What's wrong with my chart?"

"Says you were admitted with suicidal thoughts. *Suicidal inclination*—is that right?"

"That's all it says?"

Mohammed looked as though he was about to turn the screen to me, but he hesitated. "I'm really not supposed to show you."

"I know," I said evenly. "It's okay. Can you just tell me what else it says about my admittance?"

"That's really it. And there's some rule about a certain number of days being required..."

"But I wasn't suicidal...and I never said I was. I thought I told them that—it doesn't say anything in there from Mackenzie?"

Scroll, scroll. Click, click. "I don't see anything," Mohammed reported.

"Just the incoming notes from Dr. Patel?"

"That's right."

Fucking Dr. Patel, adding his own incorrect commentary to my silences. Now I was in this mess. Stuck in here for three more days *at least. Be rational*, I thought. *What action can you take* right now *to address this?*

"Thanks," I told Mohammed. "I really appreciate you looking that up for me."

"What do you mean?" he said, conspiratorially. "I didn't show you anything."

"Yeah," I said, nodding and wiping away the last of my tears. "Nothing at all."

I gave him a ghost of a smile and took a deep, therapeutic breath. Taking two laps around the ward, I readied myself to be rational and reasonable when I addressed Joanne. She had seen firsthand what an unreasonable prick the Moranster had been, and she had seemed to at least understand my perspective.

When I walked up to the nurse's station, Dr. Moran was just

closing the office door behind him to leave. I did not make eye contact but stopped purposefully in front him to stare long and hard at his name badge. He would know that I was committing his name to memory. I had make him reflect on his reckless and unprofessional behavior. I hoped he would fall asleep tonight shuddering and clinging to his medical degree while my slit gaze haunted his bedtime thoughts.

He left, and I wandered up to the nurse's station window. Yulia was on guard duty at that station and saw me holding my breath to stop from crying.

"It's okay to cry," she said kindly. "Sometimes I feel I will cry too."

"I just feel like I'll look crazy if I'm crying," I told her.

"Everybody cries in here," she said. "Even us sometimes."

I raised my eyebrows in surprise and smiled sadly as Yulia went back to filling in her Sudoku puzzle. Walking past her, I knocked on the glass of the nurse's station window to make eye contact with Joanne, who rushed out immediately.

I opened my mouth to start my explanation, but she beat me to it, apologizing in her slow even tone. "I'm so sorry. He's getting old...not very good at listening. You saw."

"Then why is he still practicing?" I said begrudgingly. "That's not what I wanted to talk to you about though. I think...I think some stuff in my chart's wrong." Damn it, my throat was already closing up. *Keep it together.*

But Joanne listened patiently through my stutters and awkward pauses as I told her where I thought I had been misunderstood, and how Dr. Patel had likely filled in my silences. "I was *not* suicidal," I emphasized, thinking even if I had been, this was not the type of facility where you would discover renewed reasons for living. "And even though an ambulance brought

171

me in, I started the chain of events that got me in here... that has to be grounds for being self-admitted, doesn't it? If I could just explain to him..."

But Joanne shook her head. "I'll put this in your chart. You're right—I don't think there's any reason to keep you here until Wednesday. You're doing fine."

My chest swelled; her validation meant everything.

Joanne continued, "Mackenzie will be here tomorrow. Tuesday too. And Mackenzie's great."

"And she's able to discharge me?" I confirmed.

"Yep."

"Great," I sighed with relief. I started to turn away but then turned back to Joanne. "Was I really rude to walk out from the office like that? I didn't mean to be—I was just really disappointed."

Joanne rolled her eyes and smirked. "I would have done the same thing."

My heart soared. It was not a final answer, but it was something to hold on to.

After getting my medical record set straight, I was hit with a tidal wave of exhaustion. I retreated back to my room to dig through my paper bag for Billie's turquoise marker and jot every miserable detail down on the legal pad that had now become my prized testament.

Venetia came in to do a contraband check, but luckily my orange juice carton and Lorna Doone's were hidden under my newspaper pile of crosswords, and the marker, already in my hand, was easy to slip under my thigh. She did not bother informing me that my giraffe and flower pot pictures were a fire hazard, probably because there was no profanity to balk at. Finally, she peered into my bathroom.

"Those scratches on the mirror were there when I got here," I told her proactively.

"I know, hon. You're fine."

"Okay, good. Just making sure."

"You writing a story or something?" she asked, tipping her chin toward my legal pad.

I prayed she did not notice the scribbles were written in ink. "Something like that."

"Glad you're staying busy," she said on her way out.

Making sure she was really gone, I settled back into a comfortable position on my back with the paper resting against my knees. I eyed the door; Venetia had left it much more open than before. I tried to ignore it but eventually got up huffily to put it back in its proper barely-ajar position. I finished my notes, flipped the pad back to the front page, and tried my hardest not to think about the Moranster's purple face with its sharp moles and wobbling jowls.

I should not have been too surprised by my encounters with either Dr. Patel or Dr. Moran. These interactions were just the latest in a long sordid catalog of lackluster mental healthcare experiences. From inconsistent diagnoses between practices to insurance battles to trying to find a therapist that jives, securing good treatment is no walk in the park. It is costly and confusing. And since few people talk about their experiences with their friends, it can be hard to pick up tribal knowledge about what to do. And even once you do start to understand the complicated process, you have to carve out the time for psychiatry appointments, the time for therapy. For the past year, I had been traveling forty-five minutes on public transit and then sitting in a waiting room for twenty minutes more just to have a fifteen minute appointment with a doctor. Then forty-five minutes back home.

The hardest for me has always been the meds. I cannot count the number of times I have been told "antidepressants aren't an exact science" and "it varies from person to person," and it is upsetting every time. When you have committed the energy to Seek Help, it is so frustrating to hear that Help will take more work. In five years, I have tried an equal number of different medications. There have been dose modifications. I have tried taking them at different times of the day. And I have tracked their side effects like it is my job while trying to work out whether each physiological or emotional change is due to the medication adjustment or because of the latest, as the professionals call it, "life event."

Are my hands sweaty because I just doubled my dose of citalopram or because that cute guy has looked at me twice now?

Is my sex drive down as a possible side effect of duloxetine or because I am just stressed about next week's big presentation?

Oh, my gums are bleeding? That's a new one.

Now I am exhausted all the time? Well, they did list fatigue as a possible side effect. Or it could just be worsening depression. Or I could simply be sleeping poorly because the neighbors like to play dubstep past midnight. Who can really say!

And that is assuming my adherence is high. Adherence means "sticking to your doctor's recommended treatment plan," and in my case, that has always meant taking my meds, every day, at a particular time. And I am *bad* at it.

But incredible solutions are being developed to many of these problems and at every step of the process. More accurate testing methods are being made. Treatment methods are becoming more standardized. Piles of data are being used to improve provider matching. Telemedicine and teletherapy are making it easier to be treated. Personalized medicine is being studied and developed. There are now dozens of quality apps that help digitally track possible side effects. And wearable technology that communicates with doctors is being created and approved by the FDA.

I try to read these stories in the news as often as possible because without them, it is easy to feel like mental health treatment is terrible and never going to improve. But every time I think that something is being implemented too slowly, too inconsistently, or too restrictively, I remember it is better than no improvement at all. A small step forward is still a forward step, and that gives me hope.

22

What The Doctor Ordered

I woke up from my snooze feeling recovered from the afternoon's disappointment, and that felt like a minor miracle. I peeled off the damp tee shirt I had fallen asleep in and swapped it out for a new one. Yanking on my least-dirty pair of socks, I stepped into the hall to check the time.

I had slept all the way through quiet hours.

According to the laminated schedule posted around the ward, we should have been having group therapy. On Sundays at 4:00 p.m., we were supposed to have a session on coping and survival skills, but when I made my way into Dayroom A, everyone was just circling word-searches with crayons or leaning back in their chairs. I guess you could call this a form of coping, a type of survival skill. There was not much healing being done in this place anyway unless you counted the treatment we gave ourselves in the form of situational friendships.

"If this was *Orange Is the New Black*, Billie would be the Russian."

We were back in the day room and assigning each other

characters like a live Buzzfeed quiz.

Billie bristled. "Who's that? She sounds mean!"

"She's like the matriarch," I explained, entering the conversation. "She makes sure all of her girls are taken care of."

"Oh, okay."

"She's mean when she has to be," Angelique explained. "And her hair is all spiky and red—that's her nickname. Red."

"Cool, I can be Red," Billie said proudly.

"Who would I be?" Angelique asked.

The room thought about it.

"I don't know. Maybe Taystee?" I offered.

"Which one's that?"

"The Black one," I said. "She's friends with Poussey and is cheerful and spirited."

"You guys think I'm cheerful?" Angelique asked, one of her usual big smiles creeping across her face.

"Course we do!" That was Nina. "Who would I be?"

Everyone went around giving their opinions. We all agreed that no one was Piper, and a few people were that one Latina woman who was always crying into the phone. Half the group said I would be Soso, probably just because I am half Asian.

But the conversation quickly transitioned to debriefing each person's session with the Moranster. We compared how much time we all had left on our sentence. Angelique was still getting out tonight, and Nina and Big Brenda were leaving tomorrow early afternoon. Billie would be too, possibly, if she continued to behave. It really was like prison.

"Behave!" Billie exclaimed. "As if the behavior they want us exhibiting is even healthy. They just want us drugged up and silent."

"I could use some drugs," Jennifer mumbled, lurching from

the side of the room. "The detoxing kind, not the bad kind."

She was clearly becoming "dope sick," as she described it; her withdrawal was starting to come in waves. The skin under her eyes was growing darker, and she looked like she could have used an entire month of sleep.

"We could ask for something if you know what you want," Billie offered.

Jennifer shook her head. "This place isn't set up for detoxing. I don't know why they sent me here." She made eye contact with Nina, and the two of them left the room together to talk.

"I'm out Tuesday morning," Mia said. "And I'll be going right to Insight."

"Oh I've been there," Angelique said. "It's great."

"Yeah, I've been before. Honestly, I wish my friends hadn't talked me into coming here," Mia complained. "I should have just gone straight there the next day. They're way better."

"What about you, C?"

I looked at Billie's well-intending expression and felt a lurch in my stomach. Everyone would be leaving before me. I would be the last one, the only one left, with no friends and no support and no real doctors.

"Didn't say," I muttered. "At least Wednesday."

From the other end of the table, Big Brenda blurted, "That's fucked up."

"Yeah," Billie agreed. "What the heck! You need to get out of here."

"I want to," I said quietly. "Really badly."

"And if you want to get out, they should let you out," Billie stated.

"I walked out of the meeting with him," I admitted, smiling just a little, "while he was still talking. I just stood up, told the nurse I was leaving because he was being stupid, and walked right out."

"Good for you!" Billie said.

"Nice," Mia said.

"Did he get mad?" Angelique asked, concerned.

"Don't know. Doesn't matter. He's not the doctor on my chart, I found out, and hopefully, I'll never have to see him again."

"Hopefully *none of us* have to see any of them again," Billie emphasized. "They're all terrible. I can't believe it that Dr. Dizon just knocked my prayer onto the ground. It's fucking despicable how they treat us. And there's no therapy happening. *Bingo* is not therapy."

I looked down on my lap and let Billie ramble on about the conditions, succumbing to my thoughts of loneliness and self-pity. More than anything, I wanted a hug. And plenty of the women here would have given me a great big hug if I had asked, but that was not the kind of hug I wanted.

The kind I wanted was the kind that felt like an answer. That made me feel safe, and like everything would be all right. An "I've got you' hug. 'I'll take care of you." When I am in one of those, I can take a deep breath and hold it inside my lungs and then exhale without it catching on the way out.

There are only two people on the planet that can make me feel like that, and as far as I know, neither one of them knows I am in here. Even if I did know their phone numbers, I would not want to tell them about this. Because if I told them how badly I needed them to come here, only to have them say "Can't, sorry. Too busy," then I think I would actually die.

I always ask for help, unless I need it so badly that the denial of it would be The End.

And here I was, thinking all of this crap, surrounded by people in much the same boat that I was drowning in, and still I felt marooned. I felt like a burden to the nurses, a burden to friends both in and out of the ward, and just burdensome to everything. For God's sake, the planet was dying, and here I was sucking up oxygen and being a general waste of space.

Every once in awhile, my mind would drift back to listening to the group's conversation, but it felt so far away. For the first time since arriving, I felt like the unhealthiest one in the bunch. It was a new level of displacement and it tasted like failure. Being in here was one thing, but feeling like I was the furthest from getting out was an entirely different tier of rock bottom. It was subterranean.

You have to understand—I am competitive. I constantly compare myself to others, whether that is performing the best, learning the quickest, or improving the most. On whatever scale it is, I feel most fulfilled at the top. It was how I behaved in high school. It spurred me to graduate with high distinction while always holding down one, two, or three student jobs. It was how I had operated during the beginning of my career, having sold my first project and being poised to be promoted early. And undoubtedly, it was part of the reason I ended up on the fifteenth floor of an adult behavioral center.

Theodore Roosevelt said that comparison is the thief of joy. And he said that before Instagram was even a twinkle in Systrom and Krieger's eyes.

If there had been a TV in the ward, I would have parked myself in front of it, just to tune everything out and give my brain a break. I considered going back to my room for *Winter's Bone*, but I knew reading would not hold my attention right now, and before long I would be reading the same sentence over and over again. What I really wanted was an iPod. Spotify. Pandora. Even Apple Music. I just wanted to soak in some indie-folk-Regina-Spektor ballad of emotion soup and pretend I was in a fucking music video. That type of commiseration sounded like just what the doctor ordered. Only I had no access to music or headphones. *And* no doctors.

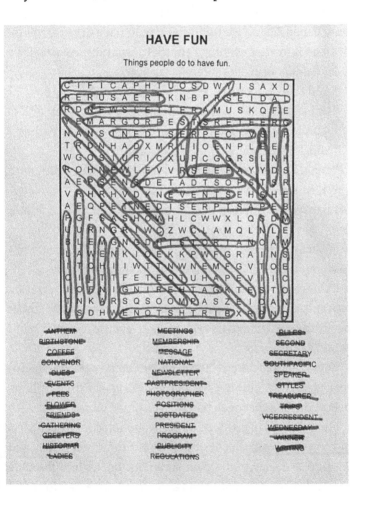

HAVE FUN

Things people do to have fun.

ANTHEM
BIRTHSTONE
COFFEE
CONVENOR
DUES
EVENTS
FEES
FLOWER
FRIENDS
GATHERING
GREETERS
HISTORIAN
LADIES

MEETINGS
MEMBERSHIP
MESSAGE
NATIONAL
NEWSLETTER
PASTPRESIDENT
PHOTOGRAPHER
POSITIONS
POSTDATED
PRESIDENT
PROGRAM
PUBLICITY
REGULATIONS

RULES
SECOND
SECRETARY
SOUTHPACIFIC
SPEAKER
STYLES
TREASURER
TRIPS
VICEPRESIDENT
WEDNESDAY
WINNER
WRITING

So as the other women in the room conversed about what they would do when they got out, what restaurant they would visit, and what stories they would tell, I selected a word search from the pile of discards and started circling the juvenile crisscrossing words. *Friends*, I circled. *Writing. Trips. Coffee.*

I was the first in line when phone hours started at 5:00 p.m. After all the people I had thought about calling, I once again only called Than. He told me I would have another visitor besides him that evening, another coworker, Anastasia. I asked him to bring me some socks, big ones.

"And I saw a doctor, finally," I reported dully.

"Oh! Did they say anything about when you can leave?"

I felt the knot rise in my throat. "Wednesday at the earliest."

"Shit," Than said.

"Yeah. He was an awful doctor, too. I'll tell you more later."

"'Kay. How are you otherwise?"

I paused, wondering how to answer. "Tell you that later too."

"Gotcha." He grew quiet on the other end of the line. "Feels like you've been in a lot longer than just three days."

"You're not kidding," I said humorlessly. The conversation was getting difficult though, so I pulled out the handy "other people are waiting to use the phone" excuse and told him I would see him soon.

When I clicked the *end* button on the compact phone, I had to look up at the ceiling to prevent the welling tears from spilling over. Why had that been hard?

I just wanted to be home so badly, bundled in a blanket on our squashy green couch, sitting in our sunny living room, and eating M&M's out of the glass jar on the too-high coffee table that our other roommate had assembled. I wanted to spend my afternoon watching Than murder aliens on some violent video game, or reading in the leather armchair that last year we had grabbed off the curb. Any of the dumb menial things I had done to pass the time on weekends prior sounded like such sweet freedoms because they happened Outside These Walls.

23

We The Special Snowflakes

Dinner was spaghetti.

Again. Same as yesterday.

I had ordered this yesterday morning.

By submitting my paper menu at breakfast.

Circled the option with crayon.

More of an oval, really.

I had thought it would be tough to fuck up spaghetti.

Did I tell you this already?

Girl sits away from everyone. Girl twists spaghetti around with plastic fork. Big fat overcooked noodles. Worm orgy in clumpy red sauce. A modern masterpiece. Girl gives up on trying to find worm orgy appetizing. Starts nibbling on corn kernels. One at a time. Picks apart the dry cookie. Sorts crumbs into two piles: edible and raisins. The raisin pile is small. Girl makes tea out of lukewarm water. Drinks it without lifting the cup, just tips the Styrofoam over a bit. It spills a little.

That was dinner.

But for the rest in the room, the atmosphere was something resembling cheerfulness. Most people had ordered the "not so bad" sloppy joes and were happily chowing and food-swapping and mingling. Closer than eavesdropping but much farther than participating, I used their conversation to anchor myself.

"I can't wait to see my boyfriend," Nina was saying. "We're gonna have amazing sex. A-ma-zing."

"I'm just excited to see my cat," Angelique admitted, grinning. "My boyfriend too. I'd probably miss him more if we could smoke in here. 'Cause he always smells like cigarettes."

"My boyfriend hates it when I smoke. But he loves me, so..." Nina shrugged mischievously.

"He only visited you once though?" Billie said.

"Lives far," Nina explained. "Plus, I don't want him to see me like this. It's disgusting."

"At least he could visit if he wanted," Angelique complained.

I did not miss my last boyfriend. But I did miss his smell. He smelled good. A stupid blue bottle of cologne. Brought it every time he visited from Pittsburgh. He was studying to be a doctor now and was hopefully learning better bedside manner.

The ex before that, the recently engaged one—he had worn cologne too. I wonder if he and his fiancé were happy. Did they want kids? Did they travel?

Jack simply smelled like deodorant and himself.

Suddenly my head was spinning. I felt sick.

Angelique was still talking. "But really," she was saying, "I miss my cat."

"They should allow animals in here," Mia stated.

Angelique's mouth made an "O," like it was the best idea she had ever heard. "Oh my God, you're right, they should. Like animal therapy!"

"Or any therapy," Billie huffed. Then she threw her plastic

fork onto her tray, where it weakly clattered. "This could be my last dinner here, everyone. After fourteen *fucking days*!"

Francine clapped and grinned her tooth-decaying grin. "We'll miss you, Billie."

"I'm going to book a hotel. Get things sorted here. Then fly back to Seattle and see my sons. See *my* cat."

"You have a cat too?" Mia asked.

"Yeah," Billie said fondly. "But I'm most excited just to be outside again."

"Right!" Nina realized. "You haven't been outside in two weeks!"

"Nope," Billie replied. "And that's ridiculous. How is a person supposed to get healthy if they're stuck inside, breathing this air, and not getting any fresh oxygen? It's crazy."

"Crazy," Big Brenda repeated.

A counselor entered the room with a clipboard. "Do-min-ee-ca?"

"You mean Angelique," Billie corrected.

Angelique turned her head. "That's me."

"Your mom's here," the counselor said in a bored tone.

"She's here?" Angelique confirmed. "It's time?"

"Yeah, get your stuff."

But Angelique barely heard her over the rest of our congratulations and go-on-get-outta-here's. Nina pretended to tear up and touched her hand to her chest.

"Don't forget about us out there."

"Forget about you guys?" Angelique gushed. "Impossible. Don't forget about *me*!"

"I don't think any of us will be forgetting anything anytime soon," Mia input.

"You have to sign your release forms," the counselor said impatiently from outside our circle.

"Give us a minute!" Billie snapped.

"Yeah, we're gonna miss her," Big Brenda said.

"Oh! That reminds me—I made you all something!" Angelique stood up and rushed out of the room, pausing at the doorway to address the counselor. "I'll be right back—one second!"

"She's so sweet," Nina cooed. "I'll miss her. I hope we can stay friends when we're all out."

"Me too," Big Brenda agreed.

I saw Mia sigh deeply and make a face somewhere between skepticism and something lighter, like hope. I understood. Out There, would people understand what we had faced In Here? And was it healthy even, to stay close with psych ward pals? The jury is still out.

"I found them, I found them," Angelique cried, slightly out of breath and holding a crinkly pile of something between her hands. "I've got one for each of you."

They were snowflakes, made out of waxy brown paper like the kind you might get a sandwich wrapped in. She had clearly folded each wobbly circle and then carefully ripped out holes to create the six-sided patterns. I had seen them hanging on her wall in her room. Each one had a tiny red oil pastel letter 'd'.

When Angelique came around to me, I hugged her awkwardly, but tightly. "Promise I'll find you on Facebook," I whispered. When I spoke, it felt like somebody else's voice coming out of my throat.

Billie clasped her snowflake with both hands, gushing, "I'll treasure it forever."

Angelique beamed.

"Ready to sign out now?" the nearly-forgotten counselor called from against the wall.

"Yeah," Angelique said with relief, accepting the clipboard. "Just sign here?"

"Yep."

"What am I supposed to sign with," Angelique said, looking cheekily at the counselor, "Crayon?"

"Do it," Mia said, handing her one from the Styrofoam cup on the table.

"God, that's perfect, isn't it?" laughed Angelique, signing in fat waxy letters. "Should I walk out with underwear on my head too?"

With final goodbyes, Angelique followed the counselor out of the dayroom. We all watched her go with a flurry of emotions.

"I hope she'll be alright out there," Billie said with melancholy. "She seems like she doesn't have too many friends to help her."

"Well, she can stay close with all of us," Nina said. Then she turned to Mia and me. "You're both local, right? And close to her age?"

"She'll need more than that though," Mia said truthfully.

We all sat on the emptiness that lingered in the room, tempered by our hopes that Angelique could return to a healthy normal. But the sobering reality was, why would she? After spending almost a week in this place, what had really changed for her? She had been a first-time ward inpatient, so maybe, *maybe*, she might now get the attention she so clearly wanted and needed from friends and family. It hurt to think about.

"Anyone else want to use the phone?" Little Brenda said, coming from outside the dayroom and breaking everyone's internal monologue.

"Oh, me!" Big Brenda said, shifting in her seat. "I gotta call my man to pick me up tomorrow."

"Ten minutes of phone time left!" a counselor yelled.

"I'M COMING!" Big Brenda bellowed.

She leapt up as quickly as her large frame would let her, and set off for the phone, leaving a comical sight for the rest of the room. As Brenda ran away from us, the back of her hospital gown flapped open, revealing her ripped paper hospital shorts and gigantic lacy black underwear. Each cheek wobbled in front of us, and the group cheered and stood in applause.

Nina pumped her fist in the air, whooping, "Run, Brenda! That's your man!"

I managed to crack a half-smile.

"I need to make a phone call too," Billie said, standing up.

I walked with her to the corner, where the counselor on duty was overseeing phone calls. Billie stood to wait in line, and I sat on the floor just inside my room, leaning against the doorframe, feeling my energy diminish by the second.

A woman I do not recognize sits down across the hall.

She is crying silently.

Billie is talking loudly.

The woman cries harder, but I am now immobile.

Billie notices.

Billie consoles her.

Billie berates the counselor.

I muster the strength to get her a cup of water.

I go to the nurse's station to get her an Ativan.

I ask for one too.

24

Visits With Ativan

Ativan hits you like a sucker punch to the gut. Before being in here, I had never had it. I had never been given any benzo—I did not even know it was a benzo until I looked it up after being released. But I could tell from the way people spoke about it in here that it was what you asked for when you did not want to feel shitty anymore. When you did not want to *feel* anymore.

Because at the dosages they were giving us, boy did it knock us out.

The tablet of Ativan I had taken my first night, from the ER nurse, had not hit me like this one was now. Maybe the dosage had been different, or maybe I had just been unconscious when I finally metabolized it, since I had gone to sleep shortly after taking it.

I have no clue how many milligrams I was given, but I can tell you that if this was force-fed to me against my will, I hands down would have bought into the old madhouse rhetoric that says conspiratorially: *if you are not actually crazy, they'll drug you until you are, just so they can imprison you forever.*

I have never done hard drugs. I have never smoked anything.

Hell, I have only been high once, during my senior spring break where my friends and I were at an Airbnb in the mountains outside Seattle. And even that was only half an edible. During that time, I sat in the trunk of the rented minivan and marveled at how pointy my fingers were. I giggled to myself. I listened to my favorite playlist with my eyes closed and ate the best Funyuns of my life.

Being on Ativan was not like that. How they portray it on TV is that the edges of your vision go fuzzy and everyone starts to talk in slower, deeper voices. Not too far off. For me, I felt like everything I was wearing was made of lead—even my skin. My tongue felt twice as large as it should have been, and my head felt too heavy to hold up. When I spoke, I could feel myself mumbling and slurring but there was nothing I could do about it. It did not make me sleepy exactly, but it did make me want to sit in a boneless, jelly-like puddle and stare blankly into space with my mouth agape.

I did feel calm though. Or at least, I did not feel anxious. Is that what calm is?

I knew it would take me ages to shuffle to Dayroom B, so I made sure to get there before 6:30 p.m. struck and visitors were allowed in. One of the staff members was brushing crumbs off the table and widely sweeping the floor. I shuffled over to one of the far tables and rested my head against the wall in order to better hold it upright. Deondra, pacing with a cold expression on her face, was just being told to leave the room.

"This room is for visitors only," the staff member was saying.

"No one's here yet," Deondra said bitingly. "I ain't hurtin' nobody!"

"Still, you have to go."

"Do I, fucker? Why ain't you tellin' that bitch too?" she said, eyeing me violently.

"I'm talking to you right now, not her."

"So you're fuckin' racist," she seethed. "Is that it? I'll kill you, I swear to God."

"Do I need to call security?"

"Man, no, you don't need to call security. You need to fuckin' leave me alone."

"I can't do that if you're in here when I'm cleaning."

"Fuck you." And she turned around and left, arms swinging at her sides.

"You can't be in here either," he tried to tell me.

From my seat against the wall, I gave him a blank stare.

"Patients with visitors only," he tried again.

"I have visitors," I slurred back. Only it sounded more like, "Iiiive visss-torss,"

He just stared, unsure of what to do, but then went back to his business.

Than came in at 6:33 p.m. and made a beeline for my table. I kept my head against the wall but sighed contentedly; just seeing his familiar face....

"Hey," said Than.

"Hey," said me.

"Brought you new socks. They're in the bag. I didn't know if 'big' meant tall or fuzzy, so I brought both."

"Thhhanks." I slurred. In fact, just assume anytime I say anything for the rest of this chapter, that it sounds like I have recently gotten my wisdom teeth pulled.

"So you saw a doctor, finally," Than prompted.

I winced. I described the encounter slowly and with each

word dragging from the last.

Than's face fell—from what I was saying and from the impaired way I was saying it.

"Yeah," I continued slowly, "And then he said the soonest I could leave was Wednesday. At the earliest."

If I had not been on Ativan, repeating that out loud to Than would have choked me up. I could tell Than was trying to keep a straight face, but it was tinged with sympathy and, even more so, barely-concealed indignation.

"If you're still in here when my family gets in for the weekend," Than said, "my mom'll be all over this place."

I smiled wryly, letting my heavy head fall onto my arm. "I'd love to see that. No doubt she'd have 'em cowering in ten."

"So really, it's Thursday at the latest. Because there's no chance she'll let them keep you here."

"Thursday at the latest," I repeated.

"What's the doctor's name?"

"Moran. In my head I call 'im the Moranster."

"Seems appropriate both ways," Than agreed.

"Yeah. I was really upset afterward. All afternoon, actually. Asked for an Ativan. Which is why I'm all..." I trailed off and wobbled my head around to illustrate my point.

My coworker Anastasia entered the room just then. Like Faith, Anastasia and I had started at our company on the same day. We both had recently been on vacation in the Mediterranean and had met up in Santorini. It was surreal to think about—just two weeks ago, we had been taking pictures together over glasses of wine at sunset.

Today, Anastasia was wearing a pretty pink dress with the same happy-but-concerned and slightly-awkward-and-unsure expression that Faith had brought yesterday. I smiled as best as I could, knowing that my eyes were barely peeking out from below my drooping eyelids.

I was not in a position to stand up to greet her, so I took her hug one-armed and from my seat. She sat between me and Than at the third edge of the table.

"This is Than," I introduced. "Than, Anastasia,"

"I remember," Anastasia said. "We met last fall."

"Oh yeah," Than said, making the connection.

"So," she said, turning to me. "How are you?"

I opened my mouth to speak but did not know where to start. Than jumped right in, filling her in on the key details.

Behind Than and Anastasia, Mia and her two visitors were deep in discussion. She had requested a list of all the medications she was on, and they were currently pouring over the papers. Like me, her head was hanging a little lower than it should have been.

I continued to converse with my visitors but was happiest to hear them talk between themselves—two people who had barely met before coming together in this makeshift visitors room for their mutual friend. Anastasia talked about work. So did Than. They updated me on the weather, and I told them about the shitty food and the dirty floors and the screaming patients. Sometimes the words would tumble out of my mouth unformed and sloppy, and other times I would only eke out a word or two.

Suddenly, a counselor walked up to our table. My head had stayed resting on my arms for their entire last hour, so I had to turn it sharply upwards just to see their face.

"You have another visitor," she said.

"Who?" I asked, both to the counselor and Than.

Than shrugged.

The counselor just added, "They're waiting."

I looked at the clock. It was 7:35 p.m. already—only twenty-five minutes left of visiting hours.

"Well, are you going to let them in?" Than said.

"Only two visitors at a time," the counselor and I said together.

"We'll leave," Anastasia said, standing up.

I wanted one of them to stay but my protest either came too slowly or never made it out of my mouth. My friends were herded out the door, and I was left to prop my head back up against the wall in order to eye the door. More than likely it was a miscommunication—no one else knew I was here, besides my team in Indianapolis and Faith, and she would have told Than she was coming.

If it *was* a miscommunication and this unknown visitor was here for someone else, then that meant my time with Than and Anastasia had just been cut short. That counselor would have hell to pay if that was the case.

Still, no one was walking through the door. Maybe the drugs were upsetting my sense of time—but no, the minute hand was creeping towards the eight. Where was this person?

My mind thought through who could possibly be about to witness me in this state. A tiny piece of me hoped it was Jack, but I know the odds of that were next to none. He would have had to 1) notice I was radio silent via text, which was unlikely because it was the weekend, and he was a terrible texter, and 2) reach out to Than, Faith or Anastasia, which was also unlikely unless he had somehow acquired one of their numbers, and 3) be free to visit me in the first place, which was the *most* unlikely because he always had a full social calendar.

But it was him. His stupid face, covered in a weekend beard, was coming through the door. It had been four weeks since I had seen him in person, and I had started forgetting his details. Five strides across the room and I was wrapped in his hug. I stood, unsteady but supported, and just breathed him in, holding tight, drinking in the familiar smell. Again, I was thankful that I was drugged at that moment, otherwise I would have started crying out of overwhelming relief, delight, confusion, you name it.

"How'd you know I was here?" I said feebly.

He looked down at me and smiled. "I know how to follow a lead."

"I look like shit," I said, thankful that at least my hair was clean and I was wearing my glasses to conceal the bags under my eyes.

"You look fine" he reassured me.

"I know I look like shit. And I'm on drugs."

He shushed me and kept hugging. "You're fine."

25

The Bed Is Not A Battlefield

I have been prescribed three different sleep aids in the past, not to mention the countless over-the-counter drowsiness medications I have tried, and I still hold that nothing will put you to sleep harder than having a tantrum. Not even great sex. I can sleep so well after a good bout of crying, and usually it's that fantastic sort of heavy, dreamless sleep, the kind where you might have only slept for an hour, but it feels like the full eight.

Scientists still do not fully understand why we need to sleep. They just know we do. Without sleep, the body begins to malfunction, starting after just one missed night. After twenty-four hours of sleep deprivation, we are as impaired as someone with a blood-alcohol content of .10—too drunk to legally drive. At forty-eight hours, the body starts to find other ways to compensate, including sudden, short blackouts. At seventy-two hours, we start to hallucinate.

At childhood sleepovers, I was always the last one to fall asleep and I could not believe that some people fell asleep within five minutes of their head hitting the pillow. And that was crazy to me! I could stare at the ceiling, thinking of nothing and everything, yawning the entire time, but still not pass out until two hours had inched by. Either my vivid, anxious imagination was keeping my mind running into the night, or else it was thoughts of how to maximize the next day, week, month. It has always been like that—sleep eluding me, dancing just out of reach until I collapse like Alice did into the rabbit hole after a maddening chase for the White Rabbit.

Then there was a time of several months where I did my best to avoid sleep in any form. My PTSD symptoms from an earlier trauma had manifested as gruesome nightmares that made every night feel like a game of Russian roulette. But even during that period, I never made it to seventy-two hours without crashing. Inevitably, no matter how anxious or scared of nightmares I was, my body's need to recharge would win out, and I would collapse for a few hours.

This toxic relationship I have had with sleep—sometimes chasing it, sometimes avoiding yet succumbing to it, and during depressive states, indulging in too much of it—made me curious. Why do we need to sleep?

The scientific community has several hypotheses but nothing concrete or definitive. There are four big theories out there (although most scientists acknowledge that the true answer is probably a combination of a few). The inactivity theory reasons that we evolved to need sleep as a survival function so we would be kept out of danger during nighttime, when our weak, clawless, fangless fleshy bodies were most vulnerable. The energy conservation theory also derides its logic from evolution, positing that sleep functions to lower our energy utilization during the part of the day when it is inefficient to hunt or gather food. The restorative theory is based on the idea that sleep gives the body a chance to restore itself, which is supported by the fact that some bodily functions like muscle growth and tissue repair happen mostly when we are asleep. Finally, there is the brain plasticity theory, which states that sleep is correlated with brain development, and that we need it in order to prevent our brain structures from turning into oatmeal.

I knew all these theories. I knew my body was built to require sleep. But it was probably something like 4:00 a.m. now—it was hard to tell, but it was still very dark, and all the loud patients must have cried themselves to sleep because there was no sobbing—and I just could not do it. I should have taken an Ambien to help me doze off, but I had already been feeling heavy from the Ativan and did not think I would need it.

The bedsheet had slid off the mat and was now crumpled at my feet so I readjusted it and tried to get comfortable. But the pillow, even folded in half, was too thin for me to comfortably sleep on my back. The mat was too thin for me to comfortably sleep on my side. And the sheet smelled too clinical for me to comfortably sleep on my stomach. So I thought about Jack.

The entire twenty minutes he had been there, Jack had kept the fingers of one hand intertwined with mine on the table. I had rested my heavy head on both our hands while he stroked my hair and listened to me babble. That small piece of human contact gently brought me out of the black ocean it felt like I was floundering in and placed me gently back onto shore.

When they called visitors hours over, I stood with him and nudged myself back against his chest, pulling his arms around me. He was tall enough—or I was short enough—that he could rest his chin on my head.

"Thanks for coming," I said, muffled by his shirt. "Sorry

for making you miss that show tonight."

"It was my choice," he said. "I wanted to come see you. They don't give too many options for visiting hours, huh?"

"Nope. You're back to Kalamazoo tomorrow?"

"You know it. But I want to see you at the show on Thursday. You better be out of here by then."

"Okay," I said, knowing I would have little say in the matter. "Thanks for coming."

"You already said that."

"Well, I'm on drugs. And I mean it." I looked away and added, "I'm sorry if I scared you."

He hugged me tighter.

We hugged twice more on the way to the locked inner ward door. Two out of the hundred I wanted. It was 8:06 p.m. when I finally got back to my room, holding the bag of new socks Than had brought me and feeling like I was made of sunshine.

I was still pretty drugged up, but I felt emotionally light enough to return to the socializing in Dayroom A. It was a party in there. Big Brenda, Small Brenda, Delilah, Francine, Mia, and a new girl, young and dark-haired, sat around the big table. Jennifer and Nina stood against the wall behind them. Mary and another new woman, Latina with box-dyed orange hair, sat at one of the smaller tables while Deondra sat alone at another. Even Gertrude and Greta were in the room.

The conversation was on talents. Turns out, Small Brenda knows five languages including Tagalog, which I learned is pronounced ta-GAH-log and not TAG-a-log, like I had always pronounced it in my head. The middle-aged orangey-blonde-haired woman told us she had been on *America's Got Talent* to sing a Mariah Carey song, but she also later admitted she was a compulsive liar so it was especially hard to believe.

Everyone seemed pretty light-hearted, considering the venue. The room was packed with all of my usual folks, plus the Saturday evening and Sunday afternoon new admits just finishing up their first day. They were easy to spot. Besides being unfamiliar to me, their eyes roved the room more than everyone else's, and they kept their arms hugged around their midriffs. For the most part, their first cocktail of drugs had not kicked in yet either, so their faces were more expressive, and the expression they wore was apprehension.

I wondered if that was how I had looked when I first got here? Then I had a worse thought—that I was no longer considered a new admit. Three days and I was now part of the established patient group. Nowhere else can you earn seniority in just a weekend.

One of the staff members came by with evening snack—cheddar popcorn again—but I pawned mine off to Nina.

"You leavin'?" Nina asked, looking disappointed. "Jennifer was just gonna teach us how to play Spades."

"Tired,'" I explained, shrugging. "The drugs."

"Ah. Well, sweet dreams!"

Back in my room, I shut the door so only a sliver of hallway light could fall through. I kept the lights off, and sockfoot-shuffled to the window, pushing the curtain aside and careful not to knock of any of my art off the windows. If I sat with my knees up to my chest, the cool air from the vent hit my calves. I leaned my head back against the wall and took a breath so deep my lungs ached.

The sunshine feeling was already wearing away. I tried to focus on all I had to look forward to. Jack's show on Thursday. Than's family visiting for the weekend. A real breeze instead of air conditioning. But all I could think was 'Wednesday at the soonest.' Three more days of this.

Fucking Dr. Moranster, with his purple skin and his moles and his jowls and his deafness.

I looked out at the dimming city. It was still light enough to see the view, fifteen floors down. If the glass in this window magically disappeared like it did for Harry Potter at the zoo, I would tumble down on top of those industrial fans and bounce into that cluster of dumpsters. Beyond that, I saw the park where the skateboarders had been earlier, and even further, the rectangles of Chicago. The green dome of a church. A sliver of the United Center. A train with one-two-three-four train cars.

With my ears so near the glass, I could hear the wind whistling outside. I wondered if anything was happening at the United Center tonight? The last time I had been there was to see Sia for my birthday last October with three friends from work—Faith and Anastasia included. I had worn a black dress with mesh cut-outs on the sides. Dark lipstick. Heeled boots. All four of us, new consultants, successful and forging our way into independent adulthood. We had danced as carefree as we knew how and shouted out the lyrics that I now recited in my head.

That track list was resonating a bit too perfectly. *Bang My Head. Breathe Me. I'm In Here. I'm Alive.* Sia has felt this feeling.

But Jack had visited. What did that mean?

No. No to that rabbit hole. It did not have to mean anything. Focus on getting out.

Please, Mackenzie, I wished. *Please let me out of here.* I looked for a star in the darkening sky but there was too much light pollution. I crawled onto my mat soon after only to wake up hours later, restless and reeling. I could not get comfortable on my side. I could not get comfortable on my back. And sleeping on my front brought the chemical smell of the sheets right up against my nostrils.

Finally, I flattened out one of my clean tee shirts, which smelled better than whatever peroxide-like detergent they used on the bedding, and found sleeping on my front much better. I fell back asleep with my feet and hands hanging from opposite sides of the bed, fingers and toes curling around the mat's end like they were holding me in place.

My brain told me there were weapons everywhere, battles everywhere. But I was on a bed, not a battlefield, and 4:00 a.m. was a time to sleep, not fight. The battles would still be there tomorrow.

IV

Ceasefire

26

How Have You Been Feeling?

I woke up again soon after to an orderly knocking on my door. This time I could see dawn through my eyelids, and I knew he was there to take my blood pressure, but it felt like I had *just* fallen back asleep, and if I moved, I would lose this perfect position. So I ignored his knocks, and after a few more, he just left.

First victory of the day. You took them where you could in here.

At 7:30 a.m., I woke up for real. Getting out of bed, I stretched everything, my back and shoulders especially, and cracked my knuckles. I rubbed my neck, focusing on the left-side knots that were payment for sleeping on my stomach. I had slept with my hair in a messy bun piled on top of my head, and so the face that reflected back at me in the bathroom looked the epitome of tousled. But I brushed my teeth, washed my face, and then let my hair down.

Well, would you look at that—a good hair day. It came down unkinked and in nice-enough waves and still smelled good even. I threw on the big grey sweater Than had brought me, yoga pants, and my purple fuzzy socks. It was still a grungy outfit, but it was exactly the type of thing I would wear on a lazy Saturday or if I was working from home, so it felt good.

Today I was going to plan my escape.

I winked at myself in the mirror.

Leaving my room, I bumped into Billie doing her morning laps.

"You walking with me today?" she said in greeting.

"For a few," I answered, joining her on her right to avoid her bad ear.

"Good. This'll be your last chance. I'm getting out today."

"Yes. You. Are."

When we passed the dayroom, I saw Nina talking to one of the new patients I had noticed last night, a girl around my age. She had a wide face, dark hair braided to a bun, and the nicest skin I had ever seen on a person up close. Nina told us her name was Daniela and that she would have breakfast with us.

On another lap, I noticed Delilah's door now had a sign with her name on it in red, uneven letters. I assumed it was because she kept walking into other people's rooms. As Billie and I walked by, I peeked in and saw her huge frame silhouetted in her dark room.

"Don't wake the bear," Billie said.

"Right," I smiled.

"The bear will probably hibernate all day."

"Probably."

"I wish I could get a decent night's sleep like her."

"You can't?" I asked.

"Hell no. Can you?"

I shrugged crookedly. "Not last night. And it's a weird kind of sleep. You know if you want, they can give you—"

But Billie sliced her hand flatly through the air. "No more drugs."

"Fair enough."

The handful of laps we had done was making me a little dizzy, so I told Billie I would see her at breakfast and returned to my room. I was less dizzy than the days before, at least, but it had never been a goal of mine to pass out before breakfast.

I laid back on my bed, staring up at the ceiling, feet crossed at the ankles and hands folded over my torso. I used to meditate in this position, first concentrating on everything I could sense and feel in my toes, my feet. Then my calves. Knees, thighs, hips, waist. Fingertips, wrists. All the way up my body until I was hyper-focused on the present instead of drowning in the past or paralyzed about the future. I sometimes wonder why they call it "mindfulness" when really, I employed it not to be full of mind but to get away from it, to be suspended in the momentary instant and make this suspension last as long as possible before having to cope with the Next Thing.

Someone knocked quietly on the door, and my eyes snapped open to find a wide-set older woman with long, thinning gray hair in the doorway. Her blue polo told me she was another counselor, but I had not seen her on the floor before.

"I'm sorry," she said. "Did I wake you?"

Based on her appearance, I had expected a throaty rasp, but her voice was surprisingly light and bell-like.

"I've been up," I assured her. "Already walked some laps this morning."

"Great, great. Well, I'm Anna. I just wanted to come in and ask how you're doing." She smiled kindly, still standing over the threshold.

"I'm fine," I said, rubbing my eyes. "I mean, I'm good."

"Great. I know you had a rough day yesterday, so I just wanted to check in on you and see how you're holding up."

I inhaled sharply. "What do you mean, you *know*?"

Anna dipped her head slightly, catching on to my suspicion. "Nothing to worry about. Joanne told me."

"Oh."

"Why don't you tell me more about yourself?"

"Um, okay. Do you want to come in? Sit down?"

"Sure, sure."

Anna moved forward enthusiastically and sat down onto the rumpled bedsheets beside me. I figured this was one of the necessary hoops I needed to jump through before they would allow me to be discharged. Prove to as many people as possible that you can be a functioning member of society! Smile. Be strategic. Tell them what they want to hear.

"So what do you want to know?" I asked her, looking right into her blue eyes as nonchalantly as I could.

"Why don't you start with how you came to be here."

"Alright," I said. I rolled my shoulders and stretched my arms over my head, like I was getting ready for a gymnastics routine. "I got here Thursday night. I came in because I was feeling really overwhelmed and I didn't feel like I was in control of myself. And I was scared, I guess, so I figured it'd be smartest for me to come somewhere safe. Then I asked someone to call 9-1-1 for me, and the ambulance picked me up and dropped me here."

Anna smiled and said nothing.

"And I guess the reason I got to that point," I went on, knowing that was going to be her follow-up prodding question, "well, there's a couple reasons. I've been pretty stressed at work. My friend killed herself a few months ago. My other friend tried to. My ex just got engaged. And I don't know, I think maybe my meds aren't working as well as they used to. I really don't know." As a period to my sentence of symptomatic causes, I shrugged.

Anna whistled, only she could not whistle so it was just a breathy 'whew.' "That sounds like a lot."

"Yeah."

"Have they changed your medication here?"

"Yep. To Cymbalta."

"Good. That's a good one."

"I think so too," I said sycophantically. "And I hope it'll work."

Another wide smile from Anna. "Well, me too. Sounds like you just came in here to get healthy."

"Yeah," I agreed, sensing my opportunity. "And I'm really hoping to get out of here soon—did Joanne tell you that? She said I can hopefully talk to Mackenzie today about it."

"We can certainly make sure you talk to her. How's that sound?"

"Sounds good."

Anna smiled a tight-lipped smile and patted her knees. "But I do want to make sure you won't be too disappointed if we find out you don't get to leave as soon as you'd like. The important thing is that you heal."

I took a deep breath in, trying to keep my voice from shaking. Crap, were my nostrils flaring?

"I know," I said evenly. "And I feel like I'm okay. Way better than Thursday."

"Great!" Anna said cheerily. "And how have you been feeling in here?"

That question could be interpreted in two ways, I thought

wryly to myself. How *have* we all been feeling? With all the pills and all the little plastic cups, it was a miracle that any of us could feel anything at all.

I looked down at my hands, away from Anna's piercing blue eyes.

"I'm just ready to get out."

27

No Chance, No Pants

8:41 a.m. and it was anarchy.

The breakfast cart was due eleven minutes ago, causing a small crowd to surround the vacant cart space adjacent to my room. It was the largest gathering of people in one place that I had seen here, and it made for a bizarre sight. We were women in all sizes, ranging from morbidly obese to plump, and puffy to skeletally skinny. Everyone had raisiny wrinkles and folds, even the youngest of us; mine were under my eyes and in the pucker of my stomach from slouching too often. We all hunched, like the hollowed-out phantoms most of us were, and most of us kept our arms bent, elbows in, hands wrung. No one was dressed in clothes that would be acceptable in public. Those of us lucky enough to have loved ones who visited us at least had pieces from our home wardrobes, but those pieces were probably the things we would wear if we were repainting a room, or binge-watching TV, or being recorded on one of those TLC shows about hoarding or strange addictions. Those without visitors were wearing layered paper gowns with maybe a hoodie to embellish the look. And we smelled. The roll-on deodorant from our toiletry bags was either not doing its job or going unused. Collectively, we were an ugly, odorous, slow-moving bunch of hags.

"What's taking so long?" Nina asked the counselor on duty, who just ignored her.

"8:30 a.m. for breakfast," said one of the Kitten-ladies.

"Of course they're late on my last day," Billie harrumphed. "They can't do anything right."

"8:30 a.m. for breakfast!"

When the cart finally came, the crowd groaned and moved in. No one shoved, but everyone was packed so tightly together that the silver doors could not swing open.

"Move back!" the counselor demanded, frustrated. "Or else how am I supposed to open it?"

Billie directed the crowd into a messy line. "One at a time," she said to us all, then turning to the staff person, seethed, "About *time*!"

I stood in line behind Deondra and said hi, but her "hi" in response was so quiet, eyes averted, that I was scared to say anything more in case I had imagined it. I took my tray and walked down the hall, careful not to spill my water or coffee, and sat down next to Nina, who was already giving the breakfast rundown to the new girl, Daniela.

"It's your first day so you'll get the house tray. The schedule's on the wall, but it's subject to change based on who comes in. What else, what else. Oh, you can't wear your street clothes 'cause that way they can find us if we run." Nina turned to me. "Am I missing anything?"

I shrugged carelessly. "Visiting hours are from 6:30 p.m. to 8:00 p.m."

Jennifer was filling out her menu sheet for the first time and asking everyone what was good.

"Or what doesn't suck," she clarified.

I looked down at my tray, sighing. Robotically, I divvied up my hot breakfast items to the quickest takers and pocketed my hot chocolate packet. To my coffee, I added a packet of sugar and then gulped both it and the lukewarm water before spearing a hard piece of honeydew melon and nibbling the corner to see if it was any riper than it seemed.

No, it was not. Firm and flavorless, just like always.

People were still filing in with their trays when the Med cart rolled in. Nina was handed her paper pill cup and water before me, and I made sure to hold the nurse's attention so she could spit out her pill before it disintegrated in her mouth.

"Up to sixty mils, huh?" Nurse Avery remarked to me.

Pretty sure that information is supposed to be confidential, I thought to myself. But I took my meds obediently and dramatically tossed the cup back into my mouth so she might not notice my even-more-dramatic eye-roll.

A week later, the outpatient psychiatrist I would see would bring me back down to thirty milligrams and tell me that places like this usually overmedicate the patients to keep us calm.

"Any sertraline?" I asked Nurse Avery.

"Sertraline?" She said confusedly, glancing back at the charts. "No, just the Cymbalta. Billie, here you go."

But Billie looked down at the cup of meds being handed to her and then held them back out to the nurse. "That's lithium. I know it is. I can't take lithium."

Avery closed her eyes, and we all watched as she considered what to do next. I guess she decided to play ball. "And why is that?"

"Seriously?" Billie spluttered. "I have a tumor. It should say that in my chart. You can't give someone with a tumor *lithium*. My doctor called and told you people—"

"Well, I'm sorry, but Dr. Moran put this in his notes and prescribed you this medication for today."

"He's not even my doctor—he can't do that."

"He's the doctor you saw yesterday, so yes he can."

"*My* doctor, the one I see in Portland who actually *listens to me*, told this place that I can't take lithium. What kind of doctors are you that would give lithium to someone with a tumor!"

As Billie's voice raised, people unashamedly stopped eating their breakfasts to watch. Billie's face turned redder and redder in frustration, and finally she marched to the nurse's station, leaving her breakfast tray mostly untouched and her pill cup full.

"Well," Mia said, "guess she won't be leaving today after all."

The nurse finished doling out the meds but my end of the table lowered their voices to gossip.

"If that's true, what she said about lithium and a tumor, then that's really fucked up," Jennifer whispered.

"Does that happen a lot?" Daniela asked, eyes wide.

"Just keep your nose down and be as cheerful as possible when they talk to you," Nina said. "Then you'll be in and out in, like, five days. Maybe a week."

"Is that how long you've been here?"

"About that, yeah. But I'm getting out today!"

I saw Jennifer's face cloud a little with Nina's announcement. This place was a carousel of people shuffling in and fading out. It was necessary to make friends to survive, but that made it all the more difficult when it was time for those friends to leave.

I realized I would miss Nina terribly. But that realization only intensified my internal urgency to get out and get out soon.

Nina swallowed a mouthful of eggs, then said, "Remind me to write down my Facebook name so everyone can find me. I have Dom's. We should all stay in touch."

"I don't have Facebook," said Little Brenda.

"Well, get one," Nina said simply. "It's real easy. Even if you don't use it all the time, you could just use it to talk to us."

"Why would I do that?" she countered, but not in a haughty way, more like a naturally argumentative way.

Nina lowered her voice again and stared Little Brenda straight in the eyes. "So we can make sure none of us ends up in here again. Ever."

I raised my empty plastic mug. "Cheers to that."

When everyone had finished eating, or at least finished pushing their food around their plate, we all cleared our trays and got ready for Activity Group. There had been no Activity Group on Friday, Saturday or Sunday, so this was my first time attending. If I had known that Activity Group was code for Sad Exercise Class, I certainly would have skipped out.

Jared was the unfortunate staff member assigned to lead Activity, and the poor guy had the fitness ability of a panda. He was overweight, wearing the standard collared uniform shirt and khaki pants, and it looked like the mere thought of exercise was making him sweat. He walked tensely toward the front of the room and turned to face the fifteen or so women he was charged with engaging. No small feat, to lead such an ugly, odorous, slow-moving, and haggish bunch.

First, Jared made us twist from side-to-side to make sure we each had enough personal space, but enough of us bumped into walls, tables, and each other that he quickly gave that up.

"Just, uh, just do what you can," he puttered. "And try not to hit each other."

We started by stretching. The room was suddenly full of thirty arms reaching for the water-stained ceiling tiles, then fifteen heads rolling around on stiff necks.

"Now bend over," said Jared, straining from the front of the room, "and try to touch your toes."

Mia, Jennifer, Nina, and I were standing in the back row of the room, which meant the four of us suddenly had a full view of one woman's open gown as she bent over to reach her hands toward her ankles. Bare old lady ass. Right in our faces at 9:00 a.m.

"Rita!" cried Nina. "Where are your underpants!"

Mia and I struggled to maintain our laughter, but soon the rest of the room was peaking over their shoulders and giggling with us.

Rita smiled slyly and stayed bent over.

"Okay, let's do twenty jumping jacks now," Jared said, starting to flap and jump, completely oblivious to what was going on in the back two rows.

And everyone looked foolish. Almost no one in the room was wearing a bra, and if we had been a more attractive, slimmer bunch, it could have been pornographic. One of Greta's boobs bounced clear out of the side of her tank top, and I saw her tuck it back in, tongue hanging out of her mouth. Francine imitated our arm movements with a doughy grin, looking like she was trying to make her wheelchair fly. But nothing was as hilarious as sixty-year-old Rita dutifully performing her exercises, bare-assed and surprisingly sly, gown flapping.

Mia and I could barely stand it. We turned our faces away and slapped the wall, completely in hysterics.

"Okay, what's so funny?" Jared asked, huffing and puffing.

"Rita is wearing no pants," Mary explained.

"What?"

"Rita," Mary pointed her out. "She has no pants on!"

"Ohh," Jared said awkwardly. "Ohhh-kay. Okay." He stepped forward and addressed Rita loudly, "Ma'am, you need to be wearing clothes to participate in this group. Tops *and* bottoms."

Rita barely slowed her birdlike jumping jacks.

"Ma'am. Rita. You need to go back to your room and get dressed."

Amongst the sniggering and chortles, Jared tried to usher Rita out of the room with wide hand movements, careful not to make bodily contact with the old lady. Rita's smile never faltered as she traipsed out of the room on the balls of her feet, light as a ballerina, happy to be the center of attention.

As laughter continued to bubble up from the rest of us, we heard Jared calling for another staff member and asking them to escort Rita back to her room. Jared came back, sheepish.

"Alright," he said. "Everyone good?"

"Just fabulous," said Mia.

"At least you didn't have to give her a shot!" Big Brenda exclaimed.

"Hey," said the orangey-blonde haired woman who had claimed to have sang for Mariah Carey. "Do you got a shot that'll make my titties bigger?"

"Yolanda, that's inappropriate," said another one of the ladies.

"She said 'titties,'" added Mary.

"If that's real," said Greta, "can I have it too?"

Mia caught my eye and smirked. "What a circus, huh?"

Jared was quickly losing control of the room, and his eyes started darting around in panic. "How about—how about we wrap up exercises and move onto Community Group?"

From the side of the room, Deondra stretched out her arm, pointed at Jared with a wink, and—I swear to God—said, "Whatever you say, Mr. Sexy Diamond Man."

I wish I could show a picture of that poor man's face. Absolutely priceless.

When I think about it, while Jared's sad excuse for a workout lacked real aerobics or cardio, there *is* a fair chance we got an ab workout from all the doubled-over laughter. We might have started the morning as a tired, hungry horde of zombies, but Activity Group had given us some life.

In terms of medicinal quality, laughter is not just some Jedi-mind-trick placebo. It's the good shit.

28

The Privilege of Being

Without exception, everyone is the protagonist of their own story. We see ourselves as the victims to our settings and the heroes who slay the dragons. There is nothing inherently wrong with that. It is simply how our narrative-oriented brains are wired to comprehend our lives.

Where it becomes a problem is when we label ourselves heroes for doing nothing. Or worse, as victims of malicious intent rather than simply victims of circumstance.

Anxiety and depression can amplify the victimhood narrative, just like any disease. "Why is this happening to me?" and "Why does everyone else get to be happy?" are questions that have often intruded my thoughts. (I will say now that my strategies for combating those intrusive thoughts include reminding myself that I am not alone in feeling that way, and connecting with others who understand and can empathize.) It's an invaluable skill to be able to think like a hero instead of like a victim.

As I looked around the room at this cast of characters, I wondered if we were all telling the same story in our heads.

Who among us saw herself as a waiting damsel, and who as a shining knight?

I had only ever seen Billie behave like a knight, but now it was as if someone had taken her armor. Having missed out on all the fun, she returned just as we were rearranging ourselves into a circle for the next session, Community Group. She took a seat immediately to Jared's right, keeping her arms crossed, chin down. Her resting expression was typically one of passionate aggravation or passionate outrage, but this look could only be described as defeat.

From the opposite side of the room, I sent her a telepathic hug. The light and laughter that had been in the room just a few minutes ago dissipated.

"Okay ladies," Jared said evenly. "Let's get started. I want us to talk about circumstances today. And to think about why we're all here today and maybe where we want to go. Does anyone want to share something?"

Everyone averted his gaze. We could already feel an oncoming heaviness, and no one felt the need to waltz into it.

He continued, "I can start. I'm here today to have this discussion with you all, and I hope that by being here today it will help me pursue my goal of helping people in my community and getting my Master's degree. Who would like to go next?"

Another pause.

"I can go next," Nina volunteered. She adjusted herself in her seat and looked around the room at our downturned faces. "Well, I guess I'm here because I'm depressed. And, you know, there's just some stuff I'm sad about and I want to be better and healthier and really deal with it or whatever. And while I'm here..." Her voice trailed off.

"While you're here, what?" Jared said.

"Go on," Billie coaxed. "You were going to say something."

"Well, I'm just trying to keep everyone cheerful," Nina murmured. "So we can all get through the day. 'Cause being here is real tough, I think, for all of us."

Jennifer patted Nina on the back and nodded seriously.

"It *is* hard, and you do," Billie said kindly.

"It's true, you do," Mia agreed, and I nodded heartily.

"Yeah," Nina continued, more quietly. "Out there, not everyone's real understanding of this kind of stuff. But it's also depressing as fuck—oops, sorry—it's real depressing in here, so I just try to keep everyone's spirits up."

My heart fluttered, and I fought the urge to get up and hold her face between my hands and tell her about how she was doing exactly that, and how much we all appreciated it. I wanted to sit next to her on a park bench or maybe near a beach on Lake Michigan and just talk about how beautiful it was to see people smiling as they roller-bladed and listened to whatever was blasting out of their earbuds. Maybe we would be able to do that after we were released. We could go eat ice cream and take a long walk to nowhere in particular and just enjoy each other's company.

Nina smiled conclusively and turned back to Jared.

"I can go now," Mary said, raising her hand. "I am here because I have had two divorces and now I have depression and I am on welfare, but it's okay because I am going to get better and I got my GED and my goal is to be able to walk on my own. I mean, *stand* on my own. Without any help from everyone, just me."

"Divorced twice?" Big Brenda said. "That's hard."

"Sounds like you're really driven to meet that goal though," encouraged Nina.

"Yes," Mary said, nodding like a wide-eyed doll, "Yes, I will."

I smiled at her. I could hear my internal pessimist trying to formulate statistics in my head, but I pushed them aside, choosing instead to focus on the simplicity of Mary's pride in this moment. She seemed so resolute, just stating her goal out loud. In this room, did the odds of that goal being met even matter?

"Shall we continue going around the room then?" Jared said, looking at Delilah next.

Delilah was wearing her glasses today and adjusted them on her nose before beginning. Her chin quivered before she began, but her voice did not hesitate at all. "Well, I don't know why I'm here. And I don't know why I'm on all these pills. But I know that I'm *still* here because no one has been able to contact my family. So that's my problem. I mean, my goal."

"Yeah, me too!" interjected Greta, her whole body moving forward.

Delilah nodded, adding, "I want to feel better too. But I don't think that'll happen from in here."

Greta nodded so fervently her chin waggled. "I need to find a home and find my family and my kids," she said.

"You have kids?" Mia asked in disbelief.

"I got two babies," Greta explained, moving her hands over her stomach. "Only they took 'em from me because they said I was being a bad mom. But they didn't say why—they just took 'em. And I got to get 'em back."

A stocky woman named Bianca interjected, "That's why I'm here. They said I had to get better or they'd take my kids away."

Jared nodded solemnly. "Who else here has kids?"

Most of the women around the room raised their hands,

including Nina, Billie, and to my surprise, the young new girl, Daniela. Every woman who raised her hand did so high up over her head. Francine lifted both arms, each hand balled in a convicted fist.

"And who is still in contact with their kids?"

Many hands lowered. Nina's stayed up, as did Daniela's and Billie's.

"I can't see my baby in here though," Daniela said. "They said it's not allowed."

"I'm so sorry, honey," Jennifer said from beside her.

Daniela shrugged in attempted ambivalence. "It's whatever."

Big Brenda cleared her throat. "I'm here 'cause I'm bipolar and maybe I've got schizophrenia. It's my, I think, maybe third time here, but every time after I leave I feel a little bit better. So that's what I hope to get from this again."

"Third time?" I heard Mia whisper under her breath. "What the hell..."

More women shared the synopses of their stories and when it came time for my turn, I glossed over everything and simply said, "Yeah, I'm sad too, and I want to feel better," and turned to Mia for her to go. Compared to some of these women's stories of eviction, homelessness, miscarriages, spousal death, and family tragedy, my own felt story pathetic and self-centered. I had no one I needed to support; no one depended on me. My responsibilities were few, and my suffering was my own. I felt weak. And incredibly privileged.

My suburban-raised, university-educated, and well-insured woes had no place in this circle. What the hell was my problem?

Jared steered the conversation forward, asking us what we

were most excited for once we "graduated."

Billie said she was looking forward to being outdoors, and feeling fresh air and sunlight. I copped out again with "better food," which earned a few laughs and nods of agreement. But Nina could barely contain her excitement.

"I'm getting out today. And I can't wait to see my boyfriend."

"Here we go again," Billie said.

"What!" Nina said, defensive but grinning. "He's great and I miss him."

"He hasn't come in to see you though," Billie pointed out.

"He's been working!"

"And what, he's always working?" Bianca accused.

"And his car broke down."

"He couldn't borrow a friend's car?" Bianca pushed.

Nina winced. "Okay, you're not gonna believe me but he also lost his license."

Billie clucked and shook her head, saying, "He should be here. You need a guy who would swim through shark-infested waters to give you a glass of lemonade."

"And have sex with you on the beach," added Little Brenda, speaking for the first time.

"Or both," I contributed.

"Yeah," Billie agreed. "Both."

But Nina's expression never faltered. "Well he's coming to pick me up today. And no matter what, I'm excited."

Jack would never swim through shark-infested waters for me, I thought, then quickly chastised myself. One: that was not fair—maybe he would. Two: it was definitely not the time to be thinking about Jack. Or sharks.

"Actions speak louder than words," sang Billie. "Just

remember that."

"Speaking of actions," Jared said, "Why don't we go around and say what we're good at. Would anybody like to start?"

"I'm good at meeting my goals," Mary piped up.

"That's great—what do you mean?"

Mary smiled docilely back at him, hands folded in her lap. "I mean I'm just good at it."

Jared moved on. "How about you," he said, motioning to Delilah. "What are you good at?"

Delilah let out a humongous shrug. "I don't know."

"How about something good about yourself?" he prodded.

Delilah tipped her head up toward the ceiling, blinking widely behind her glasses frames. "I like to sit in my room and eat the cups."

"What!" Nina burst out, laughing. "You're not supposed to eat the cups!"

Most of us were laughing or elbowing each other in the ribs; Delilah merely smiled lightly.

"Say something else!" Nina exclaimed.

"Um—okay, I got a concussion because I kept falling out of bed, but I'm good at standing back up?"

Jared looked like he wanted to laugh himself, but either he was worried about getting fired or he really was that professional, because he simply nodded, said "That's very good. Good for you," and moved on to the next person.

Mia said she was good at creating art. I said I was good at baking and PowerPoint. Billie said she was good at looking out for people. After each of us said something, the group agreed supportively and Jared said, "Good for you."

It's an apt phrase when you add a comma too. "Good, for you." For you. We could all do well for our own set of circumstances in our own stories. And I could also release my guilt. My protagonist's journey may have been less fraught than my psych ward sisters, but I was still just doing my best.

Group ended well before 10:00 a.m., and we all dispersed back to our rooms. I was just settling into that day's crossword when Caroline, the social worker, pushed my door open, knocking after the fact. She was wearing a cute, casual, blue-and-white-striped minidress. Her toned legs were on full display, and I was suddenly very aware of how prickly my own legs were.

She addressed me by my full name and I replied, "Hi."

"How are you doing today?"

Was she asking because she cared or because it was her job? I guess the two possibilities were not mutually exclusive, but it felt more like the latter.

"I'm okay," I answered. "Feeling much better. I really feel like I'm ready to leave."

"Well that's great to hear," Caroline said, hugging her clipboard. "Just as reminder, it will be up to the doctor to discharge you. You saw Dr. Moran yesterday, right?"

I bristled and hoped she did not notice my expression intensifying. "Yeah...it wasn't that helpful. But I talked to the nurse, Joanne, afterward. And I'm really looking forward to talking to Mackenzie."

"What did Joanne say?"

"Well—" I hesitated. "It didn't really feel like Dr. Moran was listening to me. It felt like he was *actively not* listening to me, and I ended up walking out. So I talked to Joanne afterward to—sort of—apologize. And she said that she would have done the same thing."

"I'm sorry," Caroline said, seeming genuine. "That sounds

really frustrating."

"It was," I said. "Especially since, like you said, he can decide when I get out of here. But so can Mackenzie, right?"

"Yep."

"So that's why I can't wait to talk to her. She'll be in today?"

"That's right."

"Great, because I'm hoping to get out today or tomorrow morning."

"We'll see what Mackenzie says," Caroline replied, with a tight-lipped smile that told me she thought Mackenzie would say *no*.

My heart starting racing again, and I breathed deeply to keep the panic at bay. "I really don't think getting out today or tomorrow is unreasonable. I've been going to group and participating. And tomorrow will be my fifth day."

"It's not about being unreasonable," Caroline said. "It's about your safety."

I wanted to tell her that it was unsafe to stay in here, where it was even more depressing and where patients were drugged into behaving like giant slugs. But I did not trust myself to say that without sass.

"It's still my fifth day tomorrow," I said carefully. "And I was a voluntary admit. And since I no longer want to be here—"

Caroline raised a perfectly manicured eyebrow. "Is that so?"

I could feel my throat closing around the scream of, "It *is* so!" but I held it in. Backpedaling, I stammered, "I just mean that I think I would be doing better back in my normal routine."

"Are you sure? Isn't your normal routine what drove you to seek help?"

"Yes, but now that I'm feeling better," I retorted, my voice starting to rise, "I really think I would be better off with my normal support system."

Caroline scribbled something down. "Can you tell me a bit more about that?"

"Absolutely," I trilled. "I live with my two best friends from college. One of them has been visiting me *every day*. My coworkers are extremely supportive, and they all know I struggle with mental illness—I'm very open about it at work."

"What about your family?"

I winced internally. I had been thinking very little about my family during my stay, and that was intentional. I did not want them to know I was here—at least not yet. I did not want my siblings to worry—the twins were only nine! I did not want my stepmom struggling to empathize with the illogical chaos that was my mental dysfunction. And I most definitely did not want my mother right now. If I asked, she would fly down in a heartbeat, like she did for my brother when his appendix brought him to the ER during his freshman year of college. But once here, I knew she would smother me in hands-on affection, and I would feel like I needed to show her results or signs of improvement. It would turn into yet another performance, and I had no energy left to perform.

Most of all, I did not want to talk to my father. When I am feeling low, I never do. We have a good relationship. He is caring and I know he loves me, but his perpetual confidence that I will always be fine can feel like a kind of indifference as if he is too distracted by everything else in his life to notice my pain. Or worse, too occupied to sufficiently care. If I called him up from this hospital at 5:00 p.m. during phone time and told him where I was, I just could not see him hopping in the car to drive the six hours to Chicago. Even if I bucked up the courage to say, "I need you," I cannot imagine he would reply, "Okay, I'm coming now." By being in the dark, he could not disappoint.

"My family is out of state."

"Ah."

"But my roommate's family is visiting this weekend," I added quickly. "And they're fantastic."

"Great, great." Caroline shifted her weight and turned towards the door. "Is there anything else?"

"Do you know what time Mackenzie will be here?"

Caroline smiled tightly again. "Should be here soon—maybe 11:00 a.m. At most, just a few hours."

"Okay."

"Okay."

And she left.

I exhaled heavily, feeling like I had just walked off a stage. I stretched out on my mattress and tried to focus my thoughts on anything besides doctors and psych wards and family, but the vertigo was so strong that all I could think of was medication. I dozed off at one point, but Billie popped her head in, startling me back awake. She said one of the patients was teaching everyone how to salsa in the dayroom, but I told her I would pass, and she left humming loudly. The last time I tried to learn to salsa was from a friend at a holiday party that past December. He had been an excellent teacher, but I had been a lousy pupil, trying too hard to make math out of the art.

Jack had been at that party. I wished I could talk to him right now to indulge in joyful memories.

I returned to the crossword I had been working on when Caroline interrupted me. It was one of those extended-clue crosswords that *The New York Times* is so fond of, where the answers eventually spell out a clever quip. I laid on my stomach with my feet crossed in the air, spinning my contraband marker between my fingers.

One Down: Five letters for 'Look that says "I'm not happy."' I scowled. S-C-O-W-L.

Three letters for 'Shelter accommodation.' I snorted and adjusted my position on the mattress. C-O-T.

Five letters for 'Bother Persistently.' Possibly an 'e' or an 'a' as the fourth letter. N-A-G A-T.

I continued my way up and down the boxes. The dull tip of the marker made me ache for a ballpoint pen, but it was worlds better than a crayon. A bit of time slid by, and I progressed slowly, distracted now and then by the sounds slipping in from the halls. My ears picked up roughened version of "Lean On Me" eking its way out of the dayroom and I capped my marker for a moment to let the music lull over me. Every voice was scratchy or airy, but blended together. The melody sounded sort of lovely. I moved to stand in my doorway and hear better, but then Yolanda broke out into a solo of "Man in the Mirror," singing obnoxiously over everyone.

I had to admit, the woman certainly had pipes.

Deondra rounded the corner and stared at me hovering in my own doorway, slowing her gait.

"I'm just listening," I explained.

She raised an eyebrow. "Listen to *this*, girl, we gotta get *out*."

"You're not wrong," I agreed.

She nodded in approval and continued her pacing. Under her breath, I heard her mutter, "What kind of hospital makes you worse instead of better. That's all I'm saying."

THE PRIVILEGE OF BEING

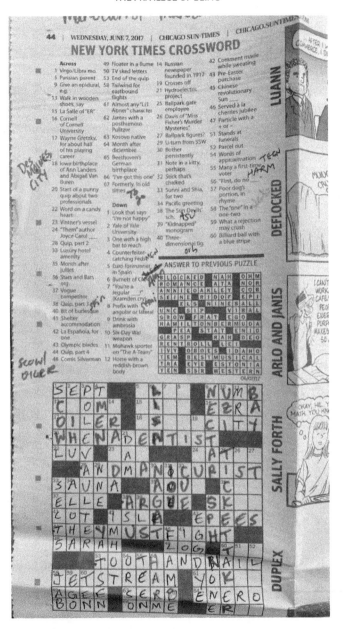

233

I picked my crossword back up and surveyed the theme clues. The answer appeared suddenly—of course it was a pun. I filled in the remaining letters and then folded up the newspaper and tossed it back in the cupboard. I tucked the marker back out of sight.

When a dentist and manicurist argue, they must argue tooth and nail.

29

When A Dentist and a Manicurist Argue

Tooth and nail.

Those had once been the weapons of choice for my personally perverted form of self-harm. There was a certain economical aspect to it that I had liked. I did not need to wield any foreign objects, no razor blades, no knives—just the sharpest pieces of my own body. Whenever I wanted to feel free or calm, or see physical manifestations of the hurt I was feeling internally, I could just rake my fingernails across my arms, my thighs, my stomach, collarbone, neck. One single deep dragging of my hand, and the hot pink lines would appear, rising in parallel on my skin.

And in fifteen minutes, the lines would be gone, with no one the wiser.

And teeth? Those came into play when I needed to stay quiet, when I was so filled with agony that it took everything I had not to scream out in anguish. I would heave empty sobs into my shoulder with my pearly whites gripping my upper arm, leaving bite marks so deep they looked like they might never fade.

Talking about self-harm is uncomfortable. Talking about all of this is uncomfortable, but self-harm especially. There is an unrelenting stigma surrounding it—that it is something only teenagers with heavy eyeliner do for attention. But like most stigmas involving mental illness, that is a dangerous generalization.

First, in *The Breakfast Club* backdrop of this world, it is not just the Allisons who are hurting themselves. It's not only a few misunderstood kids. In one international meta-analysis of fifty-two different studies, researchers found that 17 percent of adolescents had engaged in "non-suicidal self-injury" or NSSI. That's 2.5 times more students than the number that play high school football. And it is not just girls who are self-harming—35 percent are boys. Members of the LGBTQ+ community are especially prone. Bisexual girls are nearly three times more likely to self-injure than their heterosexual peers. These statistics improve as people age, but the instances do not disappear because (and now I am speaking from personal experience) it is a hard habit to break. And the impulse never fully dissipates. For me, the habit once lay dormant for two years before rearing its ugly head again after a break-up. The option is always there.

Second reason why that stigma sucks? The reasons are much more plentiful than just simply asking for attention. Many people are self-injuring behind closed doors unbeknownst to anyone, and people also self-harm to feel a sense of relief from anxiety, to have physical pain override emotional pain, or to feel *anything* in the absence of feelings in general. They might do it to feel a sense of control when everything seems so out of control, or to be punished for self-perceived faults. For some it is an addiction. For others, it is an escape hatch. Then, like me, sometimes the reason just depends on the day.

The third and most important point is this: diminishing self-inflicted harm as merely "wanting attention" suggests that wanting attention is not a valid reason for someone to self-harm. *So what* if somebody is self-harming for attention. That's a reason to *give them attention*. If somebody is *crying for help*, and you scoff at how their pain is manifesting, you are the asshole. Do not just tell them to stop, or to get over it; do not be another person in the crowd of people overlooking their pain. Not everyone has the strength to ask for help out-loud. Some can only do it by a quick, non-verbal flash of the damage.

People noticed my pink lines. Close friends. Boyfriends. I let them notice—went to them sometimes, when I was strong enough to share the pain and absolve myself. One boy would put wet washcloths over my scratch marks to soothe them. I would stand in front of him with my arms outstretched, fiercely avoiding eye contact. He would hold me as I fumed at myself, angry and ashamed for giving in to the urge. Other times, I would have to put the washcloths on myself, sitting on the floor of a bathroom, hiding from the mirror, waiting for the cold water to ease my irritated skin.

It has been hard work to get my self-harming under control, with years and years of counting how many days I could go without it, and then beating myself up when I had to start back at zero. I distinctly remember one occasion my freshman year of college when I had gone twenty-nine days—my longest streak ever—only to fuck it up on Day 30.

Today it had been over a year since I have regularly self-harmed. I say regularly because I have not completely been able to stop. Sometimes I catch myself death-gripping my own flesh, ready to rake, when I am distracted, or my thoughts are cycling out of control—like I am clinging to myself. And I still gnaw at my shoulder if I am crying really hard. But for the most part, it is no longer a habit. However, there are still some perverted associations that will always be hard to fully knock. A person will try to heat things up during sex by inflicting just a bit of pain with their fingernails, and I will shut down completely. Other times, winter weather will make my skin dry, and I will vigorously scratch the itchiness and then reel at the familiar pink lines that erupt afterwards. The deep links between scratching and shame, sadness, loneliness, and pain are still very much there.

I do hope one day that association will dissipate. Not every little scratch needs to feel like the end of the world. Sometimes, you just need to itch an itch.

30

Serf And Turf

That's one lap.
  That's another.
  And another.
  And another.
  Is that five or six now?
  Is it noon yet? Shit, it has not even been five minutes.

I was sitting in the hall, opposite the counselor on duty, counting Deondra's laps. Every time she came past me, I moved my legs farther out of her way. From here, I had an unobstructed view of the clock but I was challenging myself not to look. Everyone knows a watched clock moves more slowly.

By 11:50 a.m., Mackenzie still was not there. My nausea was subsiding for the most part, and as long as I moved slowly, the dizziness was tolerable. I thought about working on a crossword again, but the hubbub in the hallway would have made it too hard to concentrate on. Plus, I could not use my marker in full view of a staff member, and this guy on duty did not look like he would be willing to lend me his pen.

"Why aren't you in your room or the dayroom," he asked me sternly.

I looked up at him from my position on the floor, peeking at his badge. Miguel—a new face to me, just as I was a new face to him. I answered, "Just wanted some change of scenery."

"Change of scenery?" Miguel repeated, like he did not understand the phrase.

"I'm waiting for Mackenzie."

"Mackenzie?"

"Yeah, the NP."

"Oh, you mean the nurse practitioner?"

I blinked, trying not to purse my lips too obviously. "Exactly. The NP."

"Well, why don't you go back to your room. She'll come find you if she needs to talk to you."

"But *I* need to talk to *her*."

Miguel sighed dramatically. "You're really not supposed to just sit out here."

That made no sense.

I felt the corners of my face move in confusion. Miguel just continued to stare.

But it dawned on me. This was a good old-fashioned turf war. There was no rule about whether or not I was allowed to sit on the floor of this hallway—he just did not want me in "his" space. Behind the whirring computer, he was seated in his throne-like desk-chair. The surrounding linoleum was his kingdom, and I, a measly peasant, was trespassing.

Well, if he was going to play the role of indignant monarch, I would do my part to put on one hell of a jest.

"I like sitting out here—all weekend, I chatted with the other counselors—it was a good way to keep my mind off, you know, *the dark stuff.*"

Miguel said nothing. He looked away, and I considered that a sign of retreat.

I sat up straighter over my knees, peering around the wide computer screen to catch his averting gaze.

"How come you guys get name tags but we don't? *Miguel,*" I read aloud.

"Yep, that's my name."

"Do you know my name?" I challenged, knowing the answer.

"I could look it up if I needed to," he warned.

I smiled pleasantly. "You don't need to. I'm just sitting out here, waiting."

"I noticed."

"I'm pretty sure I'm allowed to do this, as long as it's not quiet hours."

Again, silence from Miguel.

"The other counselors seemed to like talking to me," I said.

"The other counselors probably weren't as busy as I am," Miguel replied, irritated. "It's quieter on the weekends here."

How could it possibly be *quieter* on the weekends? As far as I could tell, there were just as many patients in during the weekend as there were during weekdays. If anything, it was louder because there were more patients per staff members. The idea did not make sense.

"Don't you all have the same job?" I said, sweet as sugar. Then I cocked my eyebrow. "Or are you doing something else on your phone too?"

"I just meant, other counselors probably didn't mind."

"But you do," I verified. "You mind."

He looked from the computer screen, irritated. "Yeah, I mind."

I knew I could take this further, but there was nothing more to be gained. "Fine, I'll leave."

I got up just as Deondra passed by, fresh from another lap. I let her go a few paces ahead of me before following along in her wake. When I was halfway down the hall, I looked back to see Miguel slumped even lower in his chair, with his phone held horizontally six inches from his face. Probably watching porn.

I continued meandering down the ward, peeking into doors to see who was around. Most folks were napping or just looked back at me with empty stares. When I reached the nurse's station, I checked the time on that clock: 11:54 a.m. Time was a trap.

Bored and frustrated, I slid down the wall right in front of the locked door that led to the elevator bank. When Mackenzie came, she would come through there, and I would be the very first to see her.

Almost like I had willed it, the door opened, and in walked My Potential Savior. I leapt up in greeting, opening my arms to give her an enthusiastic hug before realizing that was awkward and probably not allowed.

Mackenzie reacted smoothly, giving me a calm smile and moving past me. "I'm guessing you want to talk?" she asked.

"Yes. Please."

"Let me just sign in," she replied. "I'll be with you in a moment. You can wait by the office door, if you'd like."

I waited by the same door I had lined up at to see Dr. Moran yesterday while Mackenzie strolled into the nurse's station, chit-chatting with the nurses on duty. Word spread quickly that an NP was in the ward, and soon people were lining up behind me. But I was first, and as soon as Mackenzie walked through that door, she was mine.

What was I going to say to her? That I was ready? I did not even know what 'ready' meant, but if that is what I needed to say in order to get out of here, then so be it. Could I just say that I wanted to leave? Saying I wanted In was how I ended up committing myself, so shouldn't saying that I wanted Out be enough to do the reverse?

Out was where real therapy resided. Good therapists. And good psychiatrists who focused their attention on me and wrote important things down, like what medication I should be taking. Out was where friends and family and the life I wanted to get back to existed. The pain and anguish I felt from mental illness was slight compared to what I felt from being locked in this place, away from the people who could really support me.

"Haugen, right?"

"What?" I spluttered, noticing that Mackenzie was standing right in front of me, armed with a clipboard. "Oh. Yeah. That's my last name. I mean, yeah, that's me."

"Come on in."

I felt more like a peasant than when I had been sitting in the hall with Miguel. I now had an audience with the Queen, and I was about to discover if she was benevolent. I recited a quick prayer to all the deities I could think of and stepped inside.

31

One More Cat In The Shelter

I staggered as I left the room. Had that just happened? I felt woozy, but perhaps that was the meds again, or the lack of decent sustenance for days now. That had definitely just happened, right?

None of my friends were in the line outside the office, so I started to head back to my corner of the ward, where Miguel was inevitably still glued to the phone hidden unconvincingly in his lap. I shuffled in my socks, but I *wanted* to run through the halls, banging on the floor, the ceiling tiles, all the doors.

"Yo, C!"

I turned slowly, not trusting my own limbs, to address the eager voice coming from behind me. It was Nina, dressed in her street clothes, smiling like Jesus was personally here to escort her to heaven.

"I'm leaving in *one hour*," Nina gushed giddily.

"I'm..." Dare I say it out loud?

"I'll miss you *so* much," Nina continued. "Promise we'll stay in touch?"

I nodded weakly. "Nina, guess what?"

"What!"

I whispered, "I'm getting out tomorrow."

Nina's smile threatened to crack her face in half. "Congrats, girl. The world ain't ready for us!"

She bounded off, and so I mouthed it to myself again. I am getting out tomorrow.

I had sat down in front of Mackenzie, half-prepared to make my case. But she had started the conversation by summarizing what I had told Joanne and Caroline and then had simply asked my preference. "I think you're probably okay to leave tomorrow," she had said. "Would that be okay?"

And I had answered quickly, firmly. "Yes."

She had smiled knowingly and asked if I would prefer leaving by myself and taking the bus, or waiting for a friend or family member to escort me home.

"Bus. Definitely bus." I had been prepared for this question since we had seen other patients waiting in the hallway and asked what they were waiting for. If you chose the escort, you had to wait until that person came upstairs, signed in, and filled out other forms accepting responsibility or something like that. But if you chose the bus, they gave you a prepaid bus ticket and let you leave as soon as the release paperwork was signed.

"What time would you like to leave?" was her final question.

"As soon as possible."

Mackenzie had gone into a speech on medication adherence and how I had a scheduled follow-up appointment with a psychiatrist in Uptown, but I heard almost none of it. I just nodded, beaming, trying not to cry tears of joy or start hyperventilating.

Then she dismissed me and asked me to send in the next

patient.

I was getting out tomorrow. I could not wait to tell Than tonight—I would have to wait until phone hours of course, but that was just a few hours away.

I heard Deondra's heavy footfalls and Gertrude's mumbling as they both walked their laps. When in unison, it sounded like a rhythmic chant. I neared Miguel's desk, prepared to steer clear, but then changed course to aim directly for him. Smiling wider than the Cheshire Cat, I fought the sudden urge to ruffle his hair and pinch him on the cheek. Instead, I stopped in front of him and pressed both palms into the desk, saying, "Isn't today *great*?"

Miguel looked at me like I was crazy, which, of course, I was.

"I better go see where the lunch cart is," he muttered.

"Lunchtime already," I sighed, spinning on my heels. "What a day!"

"What a day," I heard Miguel repeat under his breath.

While I waited in line, I started planning my grand return. I would call my manager, let her know I was released from the hospital and would be back online on Wednesday, the day after tomorrow. (It made no sense to return to work immediately—I would take a day to reflect first.)

Next, I would order whatever I wanted for breakfast, lunch, and dinner. I would get caffeinated coffee. Maybe I would get a massage.

No, I was not thinking big enough!

I could go to the zoo. I could go to Navy Pier. I could pay the exorbitant tourist fee and check out the view from the Sears-I-mean-Willis Tower. I could get on a plane!

Although, after whatever this hospital stay was costing me, maybe it would be smarter to stick to low-budget excursions.

Probably smart to avoid impulsive expeditions too. I could do any of a million wonderful things at home. I could stream a movie. Watch Than play video games. Bake cookies. Paint.

When Miguel came back with the lunch cart, I grabbed my tray and made a beeline for the big table. Everyone took seats around me, and the usual sound of mealtime clatter filled up the room. Big Brenda and Nina were chattering away, excited to leave.

A few women were ogling Big Brenda and clearly adjusting to her look. It was easy to understand why—Brenda's red hair was slicked back tightly, neck tattoo in full view, with dark liner drawn sharply over her lips. Everything she wore screamed Do Not Fuck With Me, which was hard to reconcile with the clumsy and bumbling woman we had gotten to know. But I suppose, give us a uniform, and we will start answering to our room numbers. Strip us down from our clothes, our make-up, our titles, and we really were just wards. So seeing Big Brenda back in her element, even if it was an element that scared me a little, was uplifting.

My news threatened to bubble out of me like a science experiment. "Guys, Mackenzie said I can get out tomorrow," I said, as nonchalantly as possible.

"Same as me, then," Mia said. "Morning?"

"Yep. Leave together?"

Mia's nod and shrug confirmed it.

"Shouldn't you two be, I don't know, more excited?" asked Jennifer. "I've been here, like, a day and already I'm dying to get out."

"Trying not to get too hopeful," I said, my smile starting to seep through. On the inside, it felt like I was vibrating.

"Yeah, that. And, you know, the pills. Keeping us leeevel,"

Mia added, drawing out the last word.

I smirked and turned to my tray. Even though I was hungry, I just picked at my meal. What I ate could have constituted a four-year-old's breakfast: the middles of the white bread to avoid the dried out crust and lukewarm hot chocolate. The lunch meat and cheese slices were room temperature and would therefore not be leaving my plate unless somebody else claimed them.

"You gonna eat that?"

Right on cue. Teri, a newer patient that we all tried to avoid, was hovering over my shoulder, pointing at my deconstructed sandwich with a stubby finger.

"Um. No. Go for it."

She did not even take it back to her plate, just picked it with her fingers and pushed it into her mouth. Then she moved onto Daniela, sitting off to the side, to ask her the same thing.

"I hate her," Nina said. "She's such a mooch."

"That's disgusting," Mia agreed, watching with fascination at the bit of bologna hanging out of Old Teri's mouth.

"Here, Teri, eat this—Oops!" As Big Brenda threw an unwanted baby carrot in Old Teri's direction, she bumped into her Styrofoam cup of juice, toppling it over.

People began throwing their napkins on the spreading orange juice spill but Nina just leaned back into her chair, looking fondly at all of us. "It wouldn't be a meal without you spilling something," she said.

"Are you ready to get out?" Jennifer asked her.

"Abso-fuckin-lutely. I'm wearing a purple thong and I've got this cute shirt on. My boyfriend and I are gonna make a baby toniiight!"

Mia and I pretended to cover our ears, and from the side of

the room, I saw Daniela smile. I turned in her direction—God, her skin was gorgeous—and was about to invite her to our table when Billie stormed into the room with the ferocity of a grizzly.

"*Listen to this*," she wailed, arms flailing in case her voice was not already getting our full collective attention. "They said I could get out today, *right*? And then they said they were gonna add lithium? Which, obviously, I can't take, because—" by way of explanation, she jabbed the air around her bad ear. "So now they're saying *I can't leave*, and it's sadistic. It's all a fucking mind game. It was a test, and I failed."

Some of the Kittens at the other table continued to shovel spoonfuls of soup into their open mouths. Those of us at the big table were quick to agree with Billie that yes, they were evil and sadistic, and yes, of course we knew you could not take lithium with a tumor.

"*AND* my kids called from Seattle," Billie continued, collapsing into an open chair. They told me—you know how I said my brother was watching my cat? Well, guess what he did!"

"What?" a few of us said.

"He gave my cat away. He just took him to the shelter and dropped him off."

"That is. Fucked. Up," Mia said.

"Seriously," I agreed. "Without even talking to you?"

"Yeah. Apparently, he just didn't want to take care of her anymore. I have been in here for *too long,* and my brother fucking gave my cat away!"

Billie was crying real tears now, and Nina leaned her head onto her shoulder and patted her back. Soon, Miguel came sauntering in to tell Billie she needed to pick up her lunch tray.

"I'm not hungry," she spoke monotonously.

"You still need to take your tray," Miguel sang

Billie's blotched face emerged from her arms, and she jerked around, eyes ablaze. "*You people can all go to hell!*"

And Miguel, with his wonderful conflict resolution skills, recoiled like he had been slapped in the face and slunk back to his desk.

32

Does Depression Hold You Back?

Everything was duller in Nina and Big Brenda's absence. They had been such an integral part of the troupe that the hall now seemed quieter without them—though the decibel level was just as eerily low and then chaotically high as always. For the most part, I was still riding the joyous wave of my discharge news, but not having Nina there to talk to, or Big Brenda to laugh with, felt disheartening. It was like they had taken a few of the world's colors with them.

Jennifer sulked most of all. Her time in the ward had only overlapped a day or so with Nina's, but they had forged a strong bond. After lunch, when Nina and Big Brenda had bid us farewell, Jennifer had returned to her room and was still there when I went to check on her in the early afternoon.

"How are you?" I asked hesitantly.

"I'm good," Jennifer answered. "How are you?"

I raised my eyebrow at her canned response. "Oh, you know, I'm just enjoying the luxurious amenities of the psych ward."

She laughed.

"You start the book yet?" I asked her, spotting *A Clockwork*

Orange at the foot of her bed.

"Yeah, but I couldn't get into it."

"I can bring you another. *Winter's Bone* reads a little more quickly."

"That would actually be great."

"I'll go grab it now," I said, backing out of her doorway.

When I returned with the new book, Jennifer handed me back *A Clockwork Orange*. "Did I hear right that you're getting out tomorrow too?" she asked.

"Yeah," I said. "Mia too."

"Wow, both of you."

"Turnover's pretty high here."

"I guess so," she said.

"Turnover's high," I repeated, tipping my head to catch her downward gaze. "That means you'll get out soon too."

"Sounds like Billie's been here for ages though"

"Just keep your head down, and you'll be out within the week," I said. "And if you're looking for more people to talk to...well, Daniela probably needs someone. And she got here around the same time as you."

Jennifer nodded, accepting my advice, and I took that as my cue to leave.

Mia was in her room as well, still working on her collages. The one I had seen yesterday had been finished and now included a ripped-out tagline from an antidepressant advert: "DOES DEPRESSION HOLD YOU BACK FROM ENJOYING YOUR LIFE?"

"Poignant," I said from the threshold. I read the top of the collage. "Mental Break? More like mental suspension."

"I'm counting down the hours until freedom," she said, squeezing more Vaseline onto her finger to paste another letter to the page.

"You and me both. Can I come in?"

"Suit yourself."

I checked the hallway for patrollers, then sat on the edge of her bed. "How are you feeling?"

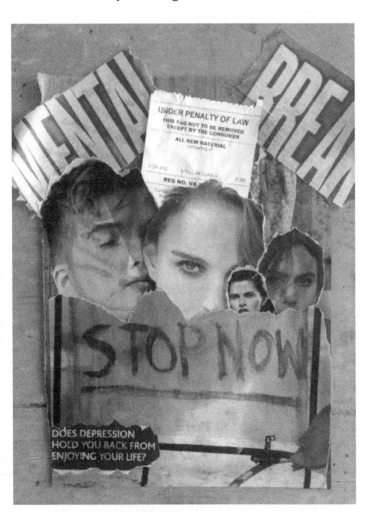

Mia looked around her room and held out her hands. "I'm twenty-three years old and this is my life. I threatened to take a bunch of pills. I get it. My friends were just—whatever."

"You're going to that other place tomorrow?"

"Yeah, that's the plan."

"Is your dad picking you up?"

"My boyfriend."

"And would he," I announced, channeling my best Billie voice, "swim through shark-infested waters to give you a glass of lemonade?"

Mia rolled her eyes. "Probably not."

"Nice that you'll have someone to cuddle with tomorrow though."

"Yeah, I guess."

"I'll just have me. The new guy that visited last night? I'm completely infatuated with him, but—it's complicated."

"I hear you."

"Yeah," I shrugged. "I've been going on dates to distract myself, and then I got ghosted by this advertising-asshat-drummer dude after, like, two months."

"That sucks. Do you miss that guy?"

I considered for a moment. "I miss his dog."

Mia snickered. "Preach. Dogs above all."

"And self-care. Living our best lives. Hashtag-YOLO."

I looked at Mia, in her Twiggy tee shirt and floral leggings. Were we real friends or just psych ward friends? I had not made many friends outside of work since moving to Chicago. In such a big city, I felt tribeless, but Mia would be fun to hang out with on a normal Friday evening. I was drawn to her attitude. Her humor. And obviously, her incredible wardrobe.

"Are you going back to work once you get out?" Mia asked.

"Yeah. I'm the only person on my workstream right now, and it's my first project so I want to finish strong."

"You like your job?"

"Love it. It's a lot, but I'm good at it."

"You love it 'cause you're good at it?"

I thought for a moment. "I don't *feel* good at it most days, but people keep telling me I am, and that always feels nice. So maybe? And also, I like feeling like I'm making a difference and helping something greater than myself move forward."

"Wow, alright."

I grinned. "But I know at the end of the day, it's just consulting. I should probably have less Kool-Aid in my diet."

"What?"

"The corporate Kool-Aid," I repeated. "Like, I shouldn't just be saying what they want me to say."

Mia told me about her job. She worked evenings, and it was a job and that was that.

"Does it ever get lonely?" I asked.

"My job? Not really. There's always people around."

"Hm, that's confusing. I still get lonely even if there's lots of people." I blinked in thought, then added, "I get less lonely when I'm busy, maybe. More lonely when I'm bored."

Mia snorted. "So this place must just make you want to kill yourself."

I smirked. "Don't say that so loudly, but yes. How are we not supposed to think about death and decay and depression when there's literally nothing else to think about?"

"Hence the art," Mia said with a flourish at her masterpiece.

"Yes, very uplifting art too," I said sarcastically.

"Can't change the color of my soul."

"Wouldn't even dream of trying."

Mia held up her collage and then announced that it was complete, and therefore time for her to take a nap. I backed out of her room and into the hallway, thinking again, real friends or psych ward friends? True friendship or situational? The question nagged at me and made me remember the last time I had misread a relationship. Within a month of moving to Chicago, I invited a girl out for donuts, during which I vomited up the greatest hits of my past and present in the hopes of forging a connection. I found out later, via letter no less, that she had felt like I had been treating her like a therapist. I could have said the same for her—hadn't we been venting together?—but it did not change the fact that learning her feelings made me feel narcissistic and embarrassed.

In this case, I would let Mia drive.

I went to Dayroom B to see if anything interesting was going on. Yolanda the lion lookalike was guarding the door. I felt her intense gaze on me as I slipped past her, feeling like an appetizing mouse. One counselor was fiddling with the radio, and Pharrell's "Happy" was again playing quietly from behind him. Mary, Francine, and Delilah were clapping along, offbeat.

Daniela was sitting in a corner with her head against the wall, staring sadly into space. I thought about going to talk to her, but the Kittens' off-rhythm clapping was making my spine curl. I tried to make eye contact with Daniela, but her attention was lightyears away from this world.

Back to pacing, I guess.

Four laps clockwise, then four laps counter-clockwise. On the laps where I walked opposite of Gertrude and Deondra, I was careful to give them a wide berth. I tried to keep my mind from wandering by counting footsteps. When I got to one thousand, I just started to count hallways, but there was so much time to think in between each corner that I lost track somewhere around twenty.

I was trying to avoid negative feelings—anger, at spending so much time in the ward without seeing a doctor or receiving substantial therapy of any kind; sadness, at being displaced from the world and not feeling the June sunshine on my face for nearly one hundred hours; and most of all, loneliness, depression's persistent specter.

So I walked, one foot in front of the other, even increasing my pace at one point to give my heart a chance at clearing one hundred beats per minute.

I wanted someone to walk next to me, in stride with me, but as soon as that idea was born, I shuddered at the thought of holding a drawn-out conversation. What if we ran out of things to talk about? We would still have to do our laps. In-room conversations had built-in escapes and were easy to end since we were not supposed to be in each other's rooms in the first place.

Wanting companionship, but not wanting all the social trappings that came with it. Was that depression or just introversion?

From the other end of the hall, Francine came barreling toward me in her wheelchair. "Group time!" she announced gummily.

"What kind of group?" I asked, wondering whether my obligations to attend were still in place, seeing as I was already approved to leave in the morning.

"Grrrrroup!" Francine said simply. "Come on, let's go."

"Alright, alright."

The two of us finished the lap, me pushing her wheelchair slowly as we dipped our heads into the rooms of alert patients along the way to let them know.

"Be there in a sec," Jennifer said from behind the pages of *Winter's Bone*.

When Francine and I arrived in the dayroom, the counselor had his back to us, but there was no mistaking those sharp corners. It was Sayed again, with his condescending voice and his swoopy hair. It would be another thirty minutes or more of him answering his own questions.

I was tempted to push Francine into the room and then bolt backwards, but she announced our presence with a noisy "helloooo!" and I lost my chance.

Endurance, I thought to myself. Maybe it will go by quickly.

"Afternoon, ladies," Sayed drawled as people continued to file into their seats. We all wrote our names in the sign-in sheet Sayed had placed next to a crayon and settled in. Jennifer and Mia sat on either side of me, and Billie took the seat next to Mia. Her face was still red and blotchy; she crossed her arms and slouched in her chair.

Holding out a thin stack of printed worksheets, Sayed explained, "Today, we're going to be talking about anger."

"How fitting," Mia mused quietly.

"Specifically," Sayed continued, "how to use anger management techniques to calm ourselves down when we're upset." The room merely blinked so he went on. "First, does anybody want to give me a definition of anger?"

Mary raised her hand and stuttered, "It's w-when you're mad."

"Can you explain more?"

"Mad," Mary repeated. "Like if someone made you *mad*."

Sayed hesitated at her juvenile response. "Riiight...anybody else?"

Jennifer, Mia, Billie, and I remained a wall of unimpressed eyeballs. Yolanda smirked from her seat at a different table but made no comment. Mary and Francine sat smiling expectantly, and a handful of others just waited for something else to happen.

Sayed plowed on. "Okay, I'll hand out these worksheets. If someone could just read the definition for me?"

Dealing with Anger

These anger management worksheets will help you to identify your anger triggers and find more effective ways to deal with anger.

What is anger?

Anger is an emotion. It is a signal that we think we are being treated unfairly.
Feelings are neither right nor wrong. **It is okay** to feel angry.
Actions can be right or wrong. **It is not okay** to hurt ourselves, others, or property when we feel angry.

So how can we deal with anger and act in healthy ways?

1) Recognize anger - know when you are angry and what makes you angry.
2) Practice positive responses - practice, practice, practice until your new positive responses become good habits.

Quick List of Ways to Cope with Anger

Walk away

Exercise

Talk to someone who you are not feeling angry with

Distract yourself

Count 10 breaths

Write about it

Come back and deal with it later when you feel calm

He splayed the two-sided photocopies onto the table, and I reached for one. The top side was titled "Dealing with Anger." A sentence below explained the worksheet's objective.

"Good God," Mia whispered. "Not again."We both looked to Jennifer to witness her first reaction to the childish worksheets. She widened her eyes at us, and we rolled ours in return.

Sayed cleared his throat. "Anyone? The definition?"

"Anger is an emotion," Mia said, loudly and forcefully. "It is a signal that we think we are being treated unfairly."

Out of the corner of my eye, I saw Deondra stand up and walk out of the room, flipping her hair over her shoulder. Now I definitely could not leave, not if Deondra had left.

Mia continued, "Feelings are neither right nor wrong. It is okay to feel angry. Actions can be right or wrong. It is not okay to hurt ourselves, others, or property when we feel angry."

Some of the words on the page were bolded, and on each emphasized word, Mia raised her voice even louder. When she finished, she dropped the page to her side.

"Great," Sayed said. "So, how can we deal with anger and act in healthy ways?"

"Are you just reading off the page?" Jennifer said, noticing the next line on the worksheet.

Sayed ignored her. "Does anyone have any ideas?"

"We could embrace the anger," Billie said stiffly.

"Yes. Are there healthy ways to do that?"

"Here's a better question. Is there a place in here where we can report if we..." Billie looked down to refer to the line and quoted, "...think we are being treated unfairly? And therefore feel angry?"

Sayed's shoulders dropped a little. "I think you'd better take that up with the doctors."

"Which doctors?" Billie said, her volume rising. "The ones who are never here?"

I jumped in before Billie could escalate much more. "You could punch a pillow," I said, remembering advice that my first grade teacher had given our class during a similar lesson.

"Yeah," Sayed said gratefully, turning to me. "What else?"

I looked down at the worksheet and picked one of the list items at random. "Exercise."

"Great, that's great. I noticed some of you like to walk laps around the ward. Does that help you feel better?"

"We do it because we're bored," Billie cried. "So we're not just sitting in bed all day, withering away."

From beside me, I heard paper crinkling and looked down to see the worksheet slowly being balled up in Mia's fist.

"I hate this," she seethed so only I could hear.

"Me too."

Sayed had other people read off from the *Quick List of Ways to Cope with Anger*. Other suggestions included *walk away*, *distract yourself*, *count ten breaths*, and *talk to someone who you are not feeling angry with*. Then he had us turn over the worksheet, where *Symptoms of Anger* were organized by physical signs, mental signs, and other signs. From where I was sitting, I thought I could spot all thirteen of the physical symptoms, including clenched jaws and red faces. In the *Other Signs* column, pacing was listed.

This gave me an idea. Quietly, I whispered to Jennifer, Mia, and Billie, "Follow my lead."

I raised my hand to point this out. "Interesting that pacing is a symptom of anger, but as you just said, it could also be a way that we cope with our anger through exercise."

"Uh-huh," Sayed said.

I cocked my head to the side, smiling slightly. "Do you think we're possibly just perpetuating our anger that way then?"

"I guess, possibly. Do you want to talk about that?"

"Not really. In fact, talking about all of this is reminding me how angry I am *right now* being here. I think I'll go..." I looked down to refer to the list on coping strategies, "...write about how angry I am. You know, as a way to cope."

Mia stood up next. "Yeah, and I think I'll 'come back and deal with it later when I feel calm.'"

My wonderful friends had caught on.

"Me too," Jennifer said. "To cope."

"And I'm just going to 'walk away,'" Billie said dramatically.

We marched out of the room, emboldened and united. On the way out, Billie threw her worksheet like a frisbee, and it fluttered to the floor near the waste basket.

Our dramatic exits were improving.

When we were a safe distance from the door, I slid down a wall and sat. "What a load of bullshit," I said.

"I can't wait to show people this one," Mia said, uncrumpling her worksheet and shaking her head. "I feel terrible. These meds..."

Jennifer yawned, grinning. "Time for another nap, I think."

"Just what the doctor ordered."

"And just what the counselors will order," I said, spotting the time. "Quiet hours next."

We dispersed to our respective rooms, and I lay satisfied on my mattress, hands resting behind my head. Fuck those condescending worksheets. And fuck those suggestions for coping with anger. Tips for coping with sadness might have been useful. Tips for coping with incompetence definitely would have been.

But then I thought about how good it felt to have the four of us walking purposefully out of that room. Taylor Swift could keep her girl squad. I had found one much better.

33

They've Got Pills For That

I never make my bed. I like to wake up in a tangle of blankets and then burrow myself into that same tangle later at night. I have always been this way, and it's one of the reasons that I preferred to sleep at my mom's house growing up, since my dad always had me make my bed. As an adult, I still forgo a comforter or duvet—just three or four blankets of various size and softness, swirled together in a colorful cloud. I never fold the blankets or bother attempting any sort of orderliness. It's my bed, and messy is the way I like it.

The only reason I tell you this is to emphasize the extremism of what I am about to say.

In the psych ward, I would get so bored that I would make and remake my bed, just to have something to do. That is what I was doing during the fourth day of quiet hours. Tucking in corners under a mattress too light and slippery to hold a sheet down. Trying to fluff a pillow that could not physically be fluffed.

Laying on top of the bed, I propped my knees up and scribbled in my notepad. My hands were stained turquoise from the marker; I had tried scrubbing the color off, but all it did was stain my bar of soap blue and make my hands smell like Dove. Again, I wished I could listen to something. The hospital should have known how easily they could lift everybody's spirits by just giving us access to our music, by letting us sift through a playlist for the perfect song and giving us a small amount of control back. Or give me an instrument. Music therapy is a thing these days, right?

Sighing, I ripped a piece of yellow paper in two. On one, I wrote "Dear Jennifer," and on the other, "Dear Billie." But I stopped there, not quite knowing what I wanted to say, just that I wanted to say something.

Quiet hours ended, but since no one announced it, and there were no clocks in each room, the ending was only made apparent by the reemergence of hallway pacers and the lack of gruff "back to your room!" barks. I saw Jennifer walking around, chewing on a cup of ice. On the next lap, she stopped to get a sip of water from the fountain, and set the Styrofoam cup down while she drank. Her elbow bumped it and it toppled over, spilling clear squares of ice across the hallway.

"Watch it," shouted a startled Jared, the counselor on duty.

"Sorry," Jennifer said, bending down to start picking up the spill.

I stood up to help, scooping the melty ice chunks into the fountain reservoir.

"Thanks," Jennifer said.

"Where did you get ice, anyway?" I asked.

"Oh, I just asked the nurses. Not being able to smoke is tough."

"I imagine every part of withdrawal is tough," I sympathized.

"It is. Especially today," she admitted, then changed her tone. "So distract me. Tell me about yourself."

"Oh," I faltered. Open ended questions are hard. "What do you want to know?"

"Anything. Where'd you go to school?"

"Minnesota."

"Did you like it?"

"Loved it. Really loved it."

"What'd you study?"

I hesitated like I always do when asked about what I studied. "I triple-majored," I said, forming my expression into a sheepish smile. "Marketing at the business school. Strategic communications in the journalism school. And psychology."

"So you're smart. What was your GPA?"

I told her.

Jennifer joked, "And I bet you know exactly which classes you didn't get A's in, don't you?"

I smiled back. "Naturally."

"I bet you got those latin honor things too?"

I smiled wider.

"Okay, Einstein, okay. You got siblings?"

We moved toward the corner of the hallway where it was dimmer and quieter. I told her about my siblings, and she told me about hers. Her face looked a lot younger when she talked about her family. She softened, then right before my eyes hardened and stiffened once again as she recalled how she had gotten hooked on dope.

"I want to get clean," she said. "But it's hard. I was trying to get clean with my boyfriend, but he got sent somewhere else. Even here, I had to say that I'm suicidal just to get committed. Then I found out they don't even have methadone, so I shouldn't be here at all."

"Have you tried getting clean in the past?"

"Yeah. But then I go back to the same environment. And it's hard to have new behavior in an old place. Nina told me something like that."

"So what's going to be different this time?" I asked. "You said your boyfriend's getting clean with you, right?"

"Yep. And hopefully we can stay clean together." Her voice trailed off, reminiscing. It was hard to tell if her thoughts were in a good place or a bad place though, so I brought her back.

"Where did you grow up," I asked, sitting down on the ground against the wall.

"Rockford, Illinois," Jennifer answered, sitting next to me. "Lots of bad shit there. It has the most violence per capita in the U.S. or something."

"Does it really?" I asked.

"Yeah, something like that."

"Well, thanks for teaching me something new."

She laughed. "And the lesson I taught you is 'don't go to Rockford'."

"Well, I grew up in rich white suburbs with money, comfort, and privilege and I still ended up here next to you." I hesitated, thinking of the point I wanted to make. "I guess I just mean...nothing's a guarantee of anything."

"You mean, it's our choices that matter most."

"Yeah."

Jennifer grimaced. "I've been on heroin for seven years. I started at your age—you said you're twenty-three? That was my choice."

"So is being in here though. You chose to come here to try and get clean. And I know this place isn't what you pictured, but you still made *that* decision and then acted upon it."

She stayed silent.

"That's not nothing," I emphasized.

A long silence again, until she spoke softly, "I really do want to stay clean this time."

"You can call me," I heard myself saying. "I can give you my number before I leave, and then anytime you're thinking about it, you can just call me. If you want."

"That'd be really cool."

"I wouldn't know any of the right things to say, but I could try. And I'd always answer the phone, no matter what."

Jennifer nodded, staring off into space. I thought our conversation was over, but then she spoke again, distant and melancholic, "We're the only sane ones, you and I."

I put my hand on top of hers, where it was resting on her knee. "Sane, insane," I said. "Who really cares? And what does it matter? We all just want to be happy and healthy."

"You know, they've got pills for that," Jennifer said.

"Even for the healthy part?"

She shrugged. "Vitamins."

I paused, preparing to voice a concern I had harbored since starting medication at seventeen. "Do you think antidepressants are just artificial happiness?"

She considered it. "I can see why you'd say that. But then you have to ask the opposite: isn't depression just artificial sadness?"

"Oh."

I liked that answer. Happiness, sadness, it was all just levels of brain chemicals.

A few yards away from us, Mia was talking to Miguel. Jennifer and I got up, and she returned to her room. I checked the clock: more than half an hour before we could start using the phone. I could pace, but I was sick of pacing. I could see if there were crayons or beads left behind in the dayroom, but I knew the odds were slim, and I did not really feel like coloring or beading anyways. I could nap, but then I would likely miss the beginning of phone hours, and I knew Than was expecting my call. Plus, I was eager to tell him that I was getting out out out out out.

In the end, I just sat in the doorframe of my room until 5:00 p.m. when people started trickling toward Jared to use the phone. I called Than, told him I was being permitted to leave in the morning, and that I would see him tonight. He let me know that both Faith and Anastasia were planning to visit too. I hit the "end" button and passed the phone off to Deondra.

"What are *you* smiling at?" she sneered.

I shrugged. "Friends."

When the dinner cart came, everyone lined up faster than usual because it was Italian Beef Sandwich Night. I took my tray to the dayroom and sat next to Daniela. I inspected my plate, lifting up the top bun first. A sizable chunk of the beef had that oil-slick shine to it, and the sole green pepper had seen better days, but it looked edible enough, apart from the fact that it was cold. I tore off the shiny bit and just ate the meat and the accompanying bowl of corn kernels. I dunked the tea bag into the lukewarm water and watched as the paper satchel quickly seeped up water and then sank below the surface.

"Mia!" Billie's voice rang out. "Feeling better?"

Mia was stomping in with her tray and slammed it on the table. "No!"

We all looked at her, blinking.

"*Miguel*," she seethed. "I asked him to write my name down

269

for the phone line but he 'doesn't do that,'" Mia drew air quotes, "and he just said he would tell me when it was time. So I go to my room to wait, right? Minding my own business. And then it's suddenly dinner time and all he says is, 'oh, I forgot about you.' No shit! That's why there's a fucking list!"

"They're all idiots," Billie said bitterly. "Lazy idiots."

"He's the worst," Mia went on. "And Jared too. Did you see him trying to exercise with us this morning? He was out of breath after, like, two jumping jacks."

"You just have to wear 'em down," I said. "Keep asking for the shit you want. Markers. Beads. Ambien. That's the only way things works in here." Listen to me. Like I was an expert.

"Some hospital," Billie said before ferociously ripping off a bite of her sandwich. "At least it's Italian Beef day."

Daniela's eyes were wide as she listened to us complain. Every move she made was minuscule and timid. I noticed her nails were long and manicured into sharp pink points that were nervously tapping her knees.

"How did group end after we all walked out?" I asked her.

She shrugged one shoulder. "Nothing else really happened."

"Yeah?" Mia verified.

"He kinda just gave up and got some crayons."

Mia scoffed. "Pathetic."

"Can I eat that?" came Old Teri's voice from over Daniela's shoulder. "Are you done with it?"

"Back off," Mia told her. "She's only had a bite."

"It's fine," Daniela said, passing Old Teri the slice of hardened cheese pizza on her plate. "I don't care."

Old Teri grabbed it without a thank you, merely inspecting the bite marks and remarking, "You have weird teeth, girl."

"Go sit over there!" Mia said exasperatedly.

270

"Suck my dick," Old Teri retorted. Still, she obeyed.

I looked down at my tray, marveling at the lack of nutritional value and flavor. This would be my last dinner here, but that fact did not demand any sort of ceremony. I saluted the crew and told them I wanted to get some reading in before visiting hours.

On my way out of the dayroom, a pop of orange caught my eye. On the backside of the anger worksheet, there had been an outline of a person, kind of like chalk at a crime scene. The instructions read, "Show on this diagram where you experience anger by shading or circling the area or writing in words." The artist had just drawn a giant orange dick on the figure's head.

I turned around and held it up. "Who drew this?" I asked curiously.

"One of the Latinas," Billie said. "The singer."

"Yolanda," I said, then grinned. "Tell her it's a great portrait of a certain president."

Billie guffawed and tucked back into her food.

I thought about how death row prisoners get to choose their last meals before they die. Photographer Henry Hargreaves created a photo series of people's last requests, and some of them are bizarre. Many ask for extravagance. Some ask for specific foods from their favorite or most familiar restaurants. The man behind the Oklahoma City bombing asked for two pints of mint chocolate chip ice cream. Another well-documented inmate asked for a single olive, pit included.

I felt like I was in the reverse situation. My unappetizing meal was the last rite before a grand return to freedom. (Though perhaps some of those death row prisoners considered dying to be a path to freedom too? Not the point.)

I was soon returning to capital-L Life, and I did not need a steak or a lobster tail to commemorate it. I would have happily eaten cardboard.

34

Teasing Tomorrow

Trying not to dwell on suicide in a psych ward is like trying not to think of an elephant when someone says "elephant" and while you are also at the zoo. The associations are everywhere. Patients threaten that they will off themselves. People complain about some aspect of the ward and say it makes them want to die. And then nurses and doctors ask constantly and callously if you feel like killing yourself. My first thought in response to that cold, abrasive question, is "No, but now that you mention it..."

Most, if not all, antidepressants come with the warning, "may cause suicidal thoughts, especially in teens and young adults." But remember this. When depression treatments are being studied in clinical phases, patients are being closely monitored for side effects. If you were being asked each and every session, "are you having suicidal thoughts?" the repeated question might suggest those very thoughts to your unconscious mind. The simple repetitive mention of suicide might make you think of suicide. What a concept.

Another thing that really gets me—when anyone says that

people who commit suicide are selfish. Fuck anyone who has ever said that. The only reason the victims of suicide lasted as long as they did is that they were thinking of the loved ones they would leave behind. They lived as long as they could and then just could not make it anymore. Trust me, people who commit suicide because of depression or chronic pain or loneliness wanted to die a long time ago. They probably wished there was a way to die without hurting anyone. Like, if they could just reverse time to have never been born, to have never forged any relationships so that they could end their life without leaving a bunch of gaping holes in the universe behind—I bet they would have done *anything* to make that an option. No one who has felt pain of such magnitude would wish more pain on anyone they love.

When I saw Than's face that night, during my last visitors hours in the ward, I again resolved to never ever kill myself. No matter how bad the feeling of hopelessness gets, I will never inflict that pain on him or any of the other people I love. They keep me anchored to this earth, *trapped* on this earth—or so it admittedly sometimes feels. But nonetheless, I am tethered. Held in place.

Faith and Anastasia visited too. We made plans for the upcoming days to meet in the office. They both seemed happier and lighter, or perhaps it was just my clearer perception since I did not have any Ativan in my system tonight, or perhaps the previous visits they had just curtailed their usual brightness for my benefit. Regardless, their cheerfulness was intoxicating. I laughed. I told them stories from the ward and made *them* laugh. And when it was just Than and me again, I started feeling a little teary-eyed.

To be fair, that might have been the sertraline withdrawal.

"What does this building look like?" I asked him.

"Big. Ugly. Think the seventies."

"Brutalist?"

He nodded. "Definitely brutal."

"I won't even look."

Than then told me that he took the day off tomorrow so he could stay home with me, and my heart tripled in size. "We can go to a café or something," he said, "If you want to write or just be back online."

"Thank you."

"And we can get whatever you want to eat."

"Thank you," I said again.

"What *do* you want to eat?"

I grinned sheepishly. "Guac? From our spot?"

"Ooookay."

"Just a big plate of guacamole!"

"Weirdo."

"Their guac is really good!"

He laughed, holding up his hands defensively. "Didn't say it wasn't!" He eyed the clock on the wall and patted his knees. "They're going to kick me out soon. I'll meet you in the lobby tomorrow morning? You think eight-ish?"

"That's my best guess," I affirmed. "I'll be hovering near the nurse's station so as soon as I'm discharged and signed out, I'll be through the door."

"Few more hours, then."

I exhaled shakily. "I can almost taste it."

Than stood up to leave. "And does it taste like guac?"

I grinned. "That, and hot, caffeinated coffee."

I cannot fully express the significance of this little conversation. Over the years, we must have had a thousand back-

and-forths about the next day's nonsense, yet that night, (and any of the other nights I have felt trapped in the present by pain), I treasured it. Buddhism and cross-stitched pillows teach us we *should* live in the present to be happy, and I try to do that too. But this is important to know: to a person who has once felt incapable of picturing a happy future, the act of talking about good things to come feels incredible. Imagining the beautiful future ahead, even if that future is the very next day, is a pillar of cognition and one of the strongest threads connecting humanity.

If being alive refers to being in the present, then living must refer to how we connect that present to a future. To me, the future is so much of the story. I am, therefore I will.

35

Hearts And Spades

"This place is worse than prison."

Jennifer, Mia, Daniela, and I were playing cards in the game room, and Jennifer was telling us about how the conditions in the ward compared to when she served time.

"Figures," Mia said, throwing in her hand.

"Worse how?" I further inquired.

Jennifer scoffed. "Worse in almost every way. Seriously. In prison, you have commissary, so you can actually get decent shit."

She was referring to the evening snacks they had just served us, which to be honest, I had not thought were half bad. I had scarfed down my bag of Goldfish crackers and apple juice like a hungry toddler at a playdate.

"And if they don't have what you want," Jennifer continued, shaking her crinkled bag of Goldfish, "You can request it and eventually it gets through."

"And the rest of the food?"

"Honestly, about the same. There was more of it in prison though, if you can believe it. And you could use the phone whenever you wanted. There were eight hours of visiting time a day. There was TV in each room—"

"*Seriously*?" Mia cried. "God, I can't believe it. I'm so bored in here."

"I know," I agreed. "I wanted an iPod. But, you know, strangulation by earbuds." I stuck out my tongue and crossed my eyes.

"Why can't we have music?" Jennifer said, placing a card onto the table. "They let us have books."

"It's not like we could kill ourselves with the written word," Mia joked.

"Isn't there something like Death by a Thousand Papercuts?" I said.

"Oh, and we were never drugged in prison," Jennifer added in retrospect. "And we went outside everyday. And there was no screaming."

"La-la-la-la!" Mia yelled. "I don't want to hear it!"

"Sorry, lady," Jennifer said. "And sorry for this too." She played her final card of the book, which meant we won the hand. Ten books to their three.

Jennifer had taught the three of us to play Spades, and we had been going for close to an hour, me and her against Mia and Daniela. I was fascinated with Daniela's long glittery nails holding her cards so delicately and gracefully. Around the room, other folks were minding their own business. Yolanda and another woman were listening to a Spanish program on the radio. A few others were coloring in the corner.

Earlier, Old Teri had taken Mia's apple while Mia had been focusing on our card game. Old Teri had then crunched noisily in Mia's ear, with a challenging smirk on her face, dancing around and taunting us. The four of us had ignored her, but eventually her taunts became wild and vocal, and the nurses injected her with a shot. The half-eaten apple was still laying sideways on the floor beside our table.

"What were you in prison for?" Daniela asked innocently, her nails tapping the table as Jennifer dealt out the next hand.

"Misuse of a credit card," Jennifer answered cavalierly. "I was there for four years. I did a lot of fucked up shit after the heroin. Every day was 'use to live and live to use,' 'cause it's a thinking disease, you know?" She continued dealing as she spoke. "Both my parents were addicts. We lived in a Winnebago—seriously. And every day was like fucking *Groundhog's Day*..."

Her voice trailed off, and we dug into our next set of cards. I organized my hand and leaned back in my seat. That was one nice thing—since there were no men here and no upstanding members of society, we could sit with our legs wide open and our stomachs pooched out comfortably. There was absolutely no reason to be self-conscious.

Daniela was massaging her breasts awkwardly. "I want my bra back."

"That makes exactly one of us," I said.

"They're sore! I just had a baby so my boobs are big."

"Ah, okay. Bra makes sense then, I guess."

"My boobs shrunk," Jennifer said, looking down at herself. "I tell you, if you want to lose weight, smoke crack."

I laughed. "Pass. Daniela, how old is your baby?"

"She's four months old now," Daniela said, a soft smile spreading over her face.

"Do you nurse her?" Jennifer asked.

"Can't," Daniela explained, "'cause the drugs. Like, antide-pressants and stuff."

279

"Postpartum?"

"I guess."

"Is that why you're here?" Mia asked.

Daniela just shrugged, eyes on her cards. "They said if I got worse, they would take the baby away."

"Jesus."

Suddenly Daniela straightened. "Can I tell you guys something?"

"'Course, honey," Jennifer said, laying down a card and collecting another book. "We're all ears."

"When I was in high school, I won this contest. For this essay I wrote."

"Cool—what'd you write about?"

"Social justice. Like, fairness. Anyway, I won, and the prize was to go to Africa."

"Oh, wow!" I exclaimed. "Which country did you go to?"

"I didn't. I was scared. It was all paid for and stuff but...I don't know."

"That's okay," Jennifer said matter-of-factly. "You're young. You had kids young so you've still got your whole life ahead of you. You can still go."

"Is that what you wanted to tell us?" I asked, watching her face carefully.

Daniela smiled. "Yeah. That I want to go to Africa. And I'm going to."

"Where in Africa?" Mia prodded. "Lots of different countries there."

"Sure, I know. But that's not as important to me. I'd like any place, probably."

"Well, I think that's really beautiful," Jennifer said. "I'd like to go somewhere too, once I'm clean. Maybe the mountains.

Or the ocean. Like you said, doesn't matter so much where, as long as it's *somewhere*."

"Right," I agreed. "Exploring somewhere new."

Daniela smiled and turned to me, looking old and young simultaneously. "Have you been to Africa?" She asked.

"I have, actually," I said, nearly whispering. "Ghana and Morocco. Last summer."

Both destinations had been part of a longer trip that made up my graduation present to myself. I had gone to cities and towns many people did not even know existed, tasted food I could barely pronounce, and met people I promised myself I would see again. I could have told these women about all of that, but I did not have the courage. My travel stories, seeped in privilege felt gratuitous and undeserved. And for all of that adventure, had it made me any happier?

I paused, quickly glancing at Jennifer, Daniela, and Mia's faces, testing the question in my mouth.

"What is it?" Jennifer asked, sensing my hesitation.

"I don't know," I faltered. "I'm just wondering... I know we're in the psych ward and all but..." and I stared down at my folded hands. "Do you think you're happy?"

No one answered right away. In the background, Yolanda and Teri started arguing in Spanish over the TV remote. Finally, Daniela spoke.

"I think I am. I don't really have a big reason not to be." She shrugged and added, "But I'm also sad, too."

"I think everyone's both," Jennifer said.

"Yeah," Mia added. "Maybe they're not even opposites."

"I just wish I could focus on the *happy* instead of all the background *sad*," I admitted. "Does that even make sense?"

"Completely," said Mia.

"Yeah," Jennifer agreed. "Like, I hate this place. But this is the best night I've had here, playing cards with you girls. And I'm happy about that."

I jabbed at her light-heartedly. "Isn't it only your second night?"

"Yeah, well, this is the best of those two."

I smiled in agreement. "Yeah, this doesn't suck."

"And," Jennifer added, turning away from us to watch Yolanda and Teri brawl over the remote, "it feels like a hell of a lot more than just two nights."

"I'll leave you my cards so you can do this every night," I told her and she smiled.

Suddenly Yolanda's body came flying toward our table. She whipped into Daniela's lap and braced herself, ready to hurl herself back at Teri, who was seething from the middle of the room with her knees bent and hands curled into claws. Someone ran for the nurses and Jennifer jumped into action, trying to talk them both down.

"Ladies!" she yelled, putting her arm in front of Yolanda.

"Fight! Shot! Fight!" someone chanted from the corner.

I stood up, back against the wall, as Mia merely leaned back in her seat, barely entertained.

A torrent of uniformed bodies came in and pinned Teri's upper body to the table. The needle went right in the upper part of her ass like a fork tine into warm butter. They continued to hold her down until her arms stopped flailing and her jaw went slack.

Mia shook her head and remarked, "I'll say it—she deserved that shot."

One last night in the cuckoo's nest, I thought to myself. Turning to Jennifer, I told her, "I'll leave you that book too.

Stay in your room—stay out of trouble."

Mia picked her hand of cards off the table, languidly thumbing through them. "What a fucking zoo."

We played another hand until the med cart rolled in. A nurse named Sheila brought me an Ambien and cup of water, bending over as I tossed cards into the middle of the table.

"Excited to be going home?" she said cheerily.

I grinned widely and sat up straighter. "*So* excited!"

"And you, Mia?"

Mia's smile was so forced it almost split her face in half, but it did the trick: Sheila kept delivering meds. I looked down at my lap, trying not to snigger.

"*So* excited," Mia mocked quietly, so Sheila would not hear. "Everything is just *super*!"

"Honestly," I addressed the table, continuing to play my hand, "Since finding out you can be discharged, has it felt like you're supposed to fake being cured? Or else they won't let you leave?"

"Yes," said Jennifer.

Mia agreed. "It's like I have to try harder in here to put on the Happy Mia show than I do out there! And being chipper is fucking exhausting."

"That could be the Ambien kicking in," Jennifer joked, playing the final card of the hand. She collected all the cards again and began to reshuffle, but I shook my head.

"Sorry, that was my last game. I'm gonna go to bed."

"Sounds good. See you in the morning, yeah?"

"Definitely. I wouldn't leave without saying goodbye."

I stood to push in my chair just as Billie came whirling into the dayroom, shouting, "Call the TV stations!"

She slid into the seat I had just vacated and paused to catch her breath before repeating, "I figured it out. Call the TV stations."

"For what?" I asked.

"To get me out of here," she explained wildly. "Tell them they're holding me against my will. Tell them all the illegal, unethical, immoral shit that's going on here and then break me out."

"You think anything will happen from that?"

Her eyes locked onto mine and she lowered her voice seriously. "You have to try."

"Billie..."

"Or else I might never get out of here." She pulled a scrap of paper from her pocket and handed it to me. It had two phone numbers written in marker. I palmed it.

"You'll call them?"

I shifted my weight uncomfortably. "I'm not sure it will do any good," I said honestly.

"But you'll try?"

I looked down at scrap of paper. "Who does these phone numbers even belong to?"

"One's my ex-husband. The other...well, just tell him that number. He'll know what to do with it."

"Okay," I said

"I talked to Dr. Eppen today," Billie said passionately, "and he said if I can just get my other doctor to call..."

"Dr. Eppen?" Mia asked. "The hot one?"

"Yeah, hot doc. Him. He said that if...if...I can't remember! So you have to just call these numbers and..."

"Okay, Billie," I said, putting my hands on her shoulders. "I'll call."

Finally she exhaled. "Great."

"Anyone else you want me to call?"

"Just those two numbers, please."

I gave Billie a hug. "Okay, I will."

Daniela and Yolanda were chittering away about their nails, guns, gangs, and catfighting—a conversation that I was socioeconomically separate from. I was nearly past the door-frame when I turned to look back.

People died every day from overdoses and cancer and freak accidents. People dealt with addiction and watched their parents pass away, and then their friends, and sometimes their own children. But people also got engaged and moved in with their significant others. They made career milestones. They found dreams and met goals and shared their accomplishments online and over coffee. They went to new continents. They fell in love.

Hearing about other people's experiences made me feel for them, but I noticed I usually reacted differently to the lows compared to the highs. I could so easily and viscerally feel other people's pain, to help them carry their suffering. But when it came to celebrating with them—it was like I saw their happiness through a pane of glass. It was alienating to see it, to see others experiencing it, while only able to feel a muted version of it. What the hell was that? If someone else's sadness could make me sad, why couldn't their happiness make me happy?

Was it selfishness? Or self-centeredness? Or the human phenomenon where, since we are only privy to our own thoughts and experiences, we give them more significance than those of other people?

Was it just comparison being the age-old thief of joy? Or was I, on some fundamental level, just truly unhappy with my own life. Perhaps no amount of goodness or joy or love or support could satisfy me.

Maybe that was the truth. When you are sad, everything can make you sadder. Your brain, seeped in misery, has a way of twisting everything into fuel for your own story of self-pity. I would love to stop the cycle—but I doubt Sayed had a worksheet for *that*.

I needed to tell these thoughts to a therapist. I need to talk these things out and have focused reflection and then be held accountable to reframing my thoughts and inner dialogue.

I tried to imagine what a therapist would say. I made a mental note to bring up Mia's earlier musing, about happiness and sadness not being opposites.

"And how do you *feel* about that?" the cynic in me imagined they would say.

I shook that stereotype out of my head. Once when I was sixteen, I had seen a therapist that told me, quote, "but what does your *heart* tell you?"

I had promptly walked out of that session and refused to see him again.

Looking around at Mia, Daniela, Jennifer, and Billie and thinking of all the others beyond this room, I tried to ask myself that question in good faith. What *was* my heart telling me, if it was telling me anything at all? I knew what my body needed. I knew what my mind needed. But what did my heart and soul need?

I thought about what made me the happiest. My friends, absolutely, even though often it feels like I cannot keep up; my mentors, and being able to proudly report back on how they had impacted me; and my younger siblings—whom I envied and was frustrated by and also loved unconditionally. Being at this hospital had been a negative experience overall, yet meeting these women had given me joy. In fact, the negativity of the ward likely magnified the joy we had found in each other.

Sadness and happiness were not opposites at all. They were more like complements.

36

Prayer

Tomorrow, I would be back to the real world, and that brought a strange type of apprehension. Excitement, muddled with unease. Anticipation, with wariness. And running through it all, doubt. Doubt for the world—would my circles still accept me now that I was stained with Commitment? And doubt in myself—could I handle a return to normalcy?

But that second question, I answered easily. If I could make it in here, I could make it out there. But simply *making it* was not really the point.

It was about more than just surviving—it was about thriving. Not stepping off the proverbial bridge was just the beginning. The next bit, the hardest bit, was never thinking about the bridge again, because there would be no room amidst all the life. When fighting suicide, we cannot just focus on saving lives. We need to focus on making lives worth living.

Finding purpose usually does the trick, but most people in their twenties, including myself, have not discovered theirs yet. Perhaps it was a matter of holding out until something clicked.

And with all these thoughts, I was already narrating my story.

"Young woman overcomes..." Overcomes what? Herself?

"Former star student battles the realities of adulthood..." More realistic, but boring.

"Teen victim grows up to become a victim once again...!" There we go with the self-victimization again.

I remember earlier that spring, Anastasia and I had gone out for sushi after work. We had been dishing about bad dates and then gushing about good ones. As we talked, we realized that what we both always felt was missing was a sense of gravity.

"A single night with a mysterious guy is almost always exciting," she had mused.

"Right, because for a night, he could be any character you imagine."

She had agreed and continued, "It's not until the second and third nights where he becomes a real person, with real ambitions and a real personality, that you either like or dislike=."

We revealed that what we both wanted from a relationship, all relationships, was to be known and felt and understood.

"Maybe dumb people have an easier time falling in love," she had joked, "because they're easier to understand. Maybe that's *why* ignorance is bliss."

"Or maybe some people just get along with everyone—and could be happy with anyone—as long as both parties put in the work."

"Could be. But I put in tons of work. Work can't fix everything."

I had considered that. I put tons of effort into my prior relationships too, even when there was nothing there to put effort toward. "Well maybe it goes back to our teenage creative writing days," I had postulated. "Always describing a better setting. Pouring out our thoughts and narrating sanctimoniously as if we can control the story. Always thinking about how the scene could unfold next and treating people like plot devices."

"That sounds bad."

"I think it *is* bad."

We had ended that conversation promising ourselves to live more in the moment. To continue adventuring, to think less about boys that did not meet our expectations, and to have fewer expectations in the first place.

But now, back in this bare hospital room, I thought about the other piece of that conversation: that all people really wanted was to be understood. To be seen and heard when they felt invisible. To feel cherished and thought of when they felt alone.

We wanted understanding from everyone—from the parent who forgot the injustice of being a teenager, to the professor we begged to extend the due date when we were overworked, to police officers who were reading the situation all wrong, to managers who treated us like we were incapable, to servers who got our lunch order wrong, to politicians we petitioned to have some humanity.

And if what we really want is understanding, was the solution to our collective misery just to help people understand? Was it *really so simple* as telling the universe what we wished for and hope that it was merciful enough to let us have it?

I played out this theory in my current setting. I did not really believe that communicating more would have solved any of the problems in the psych ward, but I did consider all of the reasons it had been hell. Could they all be rooted in the concept of not being understood?

Being admitted under incorrect classifications and held for a random number of days that no one could explain.

Seeing everyone treated the same, no matter what their cause was for being here.

Inappropriate, irresponsible, and patronizing activities sold off as therapy.

Lack of empathy from staff members.

An environment that was insufficient to every patient's needs.

Even food that our bodies did not know what to do with, or in Mia's case, that we did not eat.

The theory held.

This theory also explained why people like Billie and Jennifer and Nina and Mia had become a lifeline—because we were each going through the same experience and living the same frustrations. We understood each other.

I thought of all the conversations I would need to have tomorrow in order to reintegrate into the world. With my team at work, my friends who might have noticed I had gone radio silent over the weekend, and—oh fuck—possibly my parents?

I fell asleep with my hands clutched over my heart, trying to slow my thoughts, repeating under my breath, "Please understand me."

It was a mantra. It was a prayer.

37

You Crazy Child

An orderly took my blood pressure at 5:36 a.m. I know this because I asked him the time, and he told me precisely. From the hallway, I could see Billie already pacing, and through my window, the morning summer sun-washed Chicago in gentle gold.

"I'm leaving this morning," I told the orderly sleepily.

"Congrats," he replied, already pushing the BP machine toward the door.

"Do you know when the soonest I'll be able to go is?"

"Ask the nurses."

It had been a rhetorical question—he must have seen a hundred patients leave on a hundred different mornings, and therefore have some idea. I turned to the window and tried to go back to sleep, bunching the blankets between my legs to try finding a comfortable position. The air in the room was stale and cold, and from down the hall I continued to hear the orderly taking blood pressure measures.

Go to sleep, I thought to myself. *Then you will be out before you know it.*

But now the thoughts were flooding in, and I was fully awake. From next door, I could hear Delilah's rumbling snores. I groaned, inwardly cursing the before-dawn BP routine, and kicked the sheets off my body. Then the freezing air hit my exposed stomach and I wrenched them up again.

But today was not a day to stay in bed.

If I woke up, made myself presentable, packed, would they let me leave sooner? Might as well give it the ol' psych ward try!

Wrapping the starchy bedsheet around my body, I trudged into the bathroom and pulled the curtain-door while avoiding my reflection in the mirror. Mentally, I braced myself for the frigid water but no amount of waiting was going to make it any better or warmer. The shower nozzle made a loud "*psshhh,*" and as ice-cold drops started to spit at me, I cursed out loud and sprang back, nearly falling into the toilet. I undressed miserably and took a peek at my reflection.

It was still me. It was still the same face I had seen in mirrors and shiny surfaces all my life. She looked just like a regular person.

As I stared, a Billy Joel song wiggled into my head.

Slow down, you crazy child / you're so ambitious for a juvenile / but then if you're so smart, tell me why are you still so afraid?

I hummed quietly, still looking at myself, still undressed.

Where's the fire, what's the hurry about? / you'd better cool it off before you burn it out / you've got so much to do and only so many hours in a day

My reflection started to blur a bit, but my eyes were dry. Oh, it was just the mirror fogging.

The mirror fogging!

Glee shot through me as I realized my shower must be

293

dispersing hot water. Remembering that Billie said it was hit or miss, I leapt in.

I was no longer humming—I had fully broken into song. My own voice reverberated off the beige tiles and filled the tiny space. I had not thought of this song for years, though it had once been on my "study break" playlist on iTunes. During a few years of high school, I would use long hot showers as the middle respite within six-hour-long study sessions. The warmth of this shower stream was just as life-giving now as it had been then.

When I finished that tune, I started another, just as melodic and awash with nostalgia. I finished a whole mixtape's worth of choruses before touching the travel-size shampoo. When the water would briefly switch from hot to cold, I hugged the wall and waited it out. I was going to be so pruney and wrinkled that Than might not recognize me.

By the time I was clean, dressed, and walking beside Billie in the hallway, it was past 7:00 a.m. I was positively cheerful; yesterday had been about maintaining the façade of being "cured" but now, whenever counselors or nurses found us, there was no need to quickly slap on a false smile. My excitement was uncontainable, and I was having a hard time reigning it in so as to be sensitive to Billie's lengthened sentence.

I still had her and Jennifer's notes in my cupboard. I would make them parting gifts.

"What's the first thing you're going to do when you get out?" Billie asked me from my left.

"Go to a coffee shop to write."

"About all this?"

"Yeah," I said. "At least to start."

"That's brave of you," Billie commented. "The last thing I'd want to do is think about this place."

We passed Mia's room. She was sitting up in bed with her purple cat sweater, blinking dazedly.

"You don't look ready," Billie remarked.

Mia raised her eyebrows and said, "Oh, but I am." Then she turned to me, asking, "Do you know what time we can leave?"

"Not sure yet—I'll go ask."

I made my way to the nurse's station and rapped on the glass. Liz, one of the nice RNs with long blonde hair, traipsed up to the window.

"Hi, good morning," I said, bouncing slightly on the balls of my feet. "I'm being discharged today, and I was wondering how that happens. And when? No one's picking me up—I'm just taking the bus home."

"You won't be able to leave until whoever's in signs you out," Liz responded kindly.

"Mackenzie?" I verified. "Do you know when she'll be here?"

Liz checked her watch. "Probably not until 8:30 a.m. or 9:00 a.m.," she said. "That's pretty typical. You'll probably be all set to go after breakfast."

"After breakfast," I repeated. "Once Mackenzie gets in."

I thanked her and went back to Mia's room to give her the details.

"One final box they need to check," she complained. "Can't they just let us leave now that we're awake?"

I pretended to be shocked. "You mean you're not dying to have one last cup of decaf coffee from a plastic mug?"

"I'm *dying* to take this hospital wristband off and get the hell home!"

295

"Don't let them hear you say that word," I joked.

I skipped along, wishing a good morning to everyone I passed. Some people returned the sentiment, some ignored me, and others gave me scowls, but I did not care. One more hour, two tops, and this place would start becoming a memory.

I still needed a way to kill that time though. I manically cycled through the usual activities, watching the minute hand inch around the clock face. I even picked up a crayon and did another word search, and that is an activity that uses precisely seventeen brain cells while killing two in the process. When the breakfast cart finally rolled around, I had already swung past the nurse's station three times to see if I could spot Mackenzie in case she came in early.

At breakfast, I doled out my dry French toast sticks and hash brown triangle before poking around the fruit cup for a piece of melon ripe enough to stab. I came up empty, but I was grinning too widely to chew anyway.

"Who wants my hot chocolate packet?" I asked the crew. When no one at our table answered, I slid it to Billie. "If you don't want it, give to a new girl who comes in and needs the boost."

Mia was impatiently tapping her plasticware against the table. "Where the fuck is she? I want to leave."

"She's probably almost here," I said.

"I just want to take a nap in my own bed," Mia droned.

"The nurses said after breakfast."

"Well, breakfast is here," she stated irritably. "So now it's after breakfast."

"You want to go check with me?" I asked. "I'm not going to eat any of this fruit."

Mia and I walked together to return our trays to the silver

cart. I slid mine into its shelf and nodded in satisfaction.

"Can't wait to get an actual meal today," Mia said, sliding her tray in above mine.

"And actual caffeine."

"God, yes," Mia moaned, her eyes rolling back into her head. "Rich arabica in my *veins*."

"To be received intravenously, huh?"

"I don't care how it gets inside me," Mia said as we pulled up to the nurse's station window, "as long as it does."

"Well," I muttered under my breath as we pulled up to the nurse's station window, "no espresso enema for me, thanks."

Mia planted her feet in front of the window and knocked firmly. Liz made eye contact with us from the other side of the glass and held up a finger, but Mia spoke loudly through the glass, "When can we leave?"

Liz opened her mouth as if to shout back, but closed it and finished logging whatever she was entering into the computer. Then she calmly opened the door and smiled at us.

"Mackenzie just told us she'd be here in about half an hour," Liz said.

I could feel Mia's protest powering up inside her, but I cut her off before she could shout. "Is there any paperwork we'll need to fill out that we could get started on?" I asked. "Or could we at least get our things back? Like our phones and stuff?"

"Sure, of course," Liz answered pleasantly. She went back into the nurse's station to get the key to the contraband closet. From behind her back, Mia batted her eyelashes and mouthed, "Sure, of course."

A counselor whose badge read "Calvin" took the closet keys from Liz and led us around the corner. I recognized him as

297

the counselor who had taken my blood pressure that very first morning—a lifetime ago. He fumbled with the keys and tried what seemed like every last one on the ring before the door finally swung open.

"Okay... what are your room numbers?" Calvin asked us, scanning the shelves of brown paper bags and plastic bins. "Wait, they're here by last name. What are your last names?"

Mia and I peeked around his torso so we could just point out the bags with our belongings.

"Am I supposed to just let them take everything now?" Calvin called out to Liz, poking his head out of the closet room.

We heard her faintly reply, "Yeah—it just has to stay in the closet or near the nurse's station."

"You heard the lady."

Calvin plucked our bags from the shelves but did not hand them to us, instead reaching into our bags to give us our belongings item by item.

"Two shoes," he said, handing me my sneakers. "Phone. Phone charger."

"I can just take the bag..." I said, knowing the last item was my bra.

But Calvin pulled it out of the bag anyway and handed it to me. I did not make eye contact, just in case he was staring at my tee shirt or grinning waggishly.

"Thanks," I mumbled, taking my shoes in one hand and rolling my bra up into the hem of my tee shirt with the other. Awkwardly, I tapped the home button on my phone but—as I figured it would be—it was dead. In addition to the fact that it's battery had been draining for five days, it also had not been holding charge well for the past few months, which is why I had had my charging cable in my pocket. "Can I charge my phone? So I can look up transportation and stuff?"

"Sure," Calvin said, handing Mia her things item by item as well. "Just make sure you leave it in here."

I plugged it in and then scuttled back to my room with my contraband clothing. Sitting on the bed, back to the door, I pulled my arms through my tee shirt so it slung around my neck and then fastened my bra and pulled on the straps and then the tee shirt once again. I unlaced my shoes and slipped my feet in, marveling at the sensation of wearing shoes for the first time in five days. I stood and wiggled my toes.

Barefoot is preferable, but at this moment I wanted nothing more than to hit the pavement and sprint. I have never run more than three consecutive miles in my life, but I bet I could conquer that distance home without stopping if it meant I could leave this very second.

I would make sure I was raring to go the very second Mackenzie arrived. Ready and get set.

I tucked every worksheet and scrap of notepaper into my bulky grocery bags and then gathered them in my arms. I walked out of room 1525 without a moment's consideration.

Back at the nurse's station, I dropped my bags and camped out ostentatiously beside the counselor on duty. I was giddy. I was wriggling. I sat on the ground with my back against the wall, trying to sit as still as possible, but my fingers continued to skitter across my thighs.

Then I remembered Jennifer and Billie's letters. I pulled them out from where they were tucked into a bag and flattened out the wrinkles, rereading both.

"Will you watch my stuff for me?" I asked the counselor.

Without waiting for an answer, I took off down the hall to Jennifer's room. She was not there—probably still in the dayroom from breakfast—so I placed the note at the foot of her made bed where I knew she would see it. Backing out, I did the same in Billie's room. Where was everybody?

I heard percussive voices from Dayroom B and followed the sounds. Mia was sitting slumped in a chair, watching Yolanda and Teri argue wildly in Spanish.

"I don't know what they're saying," I said, sitting next to Jennifer.

"Want to guess?"

"They're talking about their kids," Daniela translated.

"And arguing?" I asked.

Daniela shrugged.

"Come on," I coaxed, watching Yolanda lunge forward. "You're editing—what are they really saying?"

Daniela smiled shyly but Mia sighed loudly before she could answer.

"I can't believe this," Mia moaned. "We're going to end up getting stuck here until the afternoon. Basically a whole 'nother day."

"At least we're never short on entertainment," I said sarcastically.

"This is stupid," Mia said, motioning to the two women who looked ready to scratch each other's eyes out. "Ladies, stop yelling! Don't you know it's a new day for feminism?"

"Don't think they got that memo," Jennifer said.

I tapped Mia on the shoulder. "It has to be close to a half hour. They said Mackenzie would be here by now—want to go check again?"

"Sure—it's not like they would come get us to let us know. I'm just going to grab my stuff. Meet you there."

I turned to Daniela and Jennifer, suddenly realizing this

could be the last time I ever see them. I only met them two days ago. Less than forty-eight hours.

"Good luck," I said lamely, giving them each a tight hug and hoping that did a better job of communicating what I felt.

"Bye," said Daniela.

Jennifer inhaled deeply before replying, "Stay fierce."

Then Mia and I stalked out of the dayroom and headed down opposite halls. It felt bizarre to be wearing shoes in these corridors, and even weirder to be wearing a bra. I did notice that I automatically stood straighter though.

Rounding the corner, I saw her. Mackenzie was signing in at the nurse's station, halo and all.

"Mackenzie!" I shouted, so loudly that she seemed momentarily frightened until she saw it was me.

"One minute," Mackenzie said drowsily. "I'll be right with you."

I took the opportunity to get Mia from her room. "She's here!" I shout-whispered.

"Finally," Mia said, clasping her hands together in a mock prayer of thanks.

My heart was accelerating again. I felt light-headed again.

Mia and I hovered around Mackenzie awkwardly, both of us with our bags at our ankles, as she made small talk with the nurses. We were entirely unsure of what actually needed to be done before we could leave. Did Mackenzie have to look into our pupils to see if she could spot suicidal thoughts? Perhaps she needed to take our blood pressure one final goddamn time?

Finally Mackenzie's attention was on us.

"How are you feeling this morning?" she asked us both, in an overly professional manner that suggested it was a diagnostic question and not a casual one.

"Fantastic," I responded. "Ready to leave."

"Same," Mia said. "Ready."

"Great. Well, there's just a few things I need to verify with each of you. Then a couple forms to sign. Then you'll be on your way." She turned to address me first. "You have an appointment with Dr. Tsao in one week that you committed to attending."

"Yep. All good."

"And you are currently taking sixty milligrams of duloxetine and will continue doing so."

"Yep."

"And you have no desire to harm yourself or others."

"Correct," I said, emphasizing both syllables.

"Great. Well, Liz will get you the rest of the paperwork," Mackenzie pointed her thumb at Liz who was standing behind her. "Mia, if you and I could just talk over here for a second..."

I stepped toward Liz who was holding two plain-looking envelopes, one stuffed full of papers and one nearly empty. She handed them both to me.

"This one's a summary of the treatment you got here," she explained, pointing at the fat envelope, "as well as some other information and numbers you can call. It's got your bus ticket in here too. It's also got a seven day prescription for the medication we prescribed you here."

"Does it have the side effect information? Or information on that medication?"

Liz blinked. "No... but we can print it out if you'd like it?"

I shook my head hurriedly, looking at the clock and realizing with a jolt that Than had probably been downstairs waiting for over half an hour now. I hoped he had remembered to bring himself a book. "It's okay, I'll just Google it at home."

Liz nodded. "Alright, easy enough." Next she pointed at the thinner envelope. "This is just a quick survey about your time here. If you could fill it out now, then you'll be good to go!"

I pulled the survey out and saw the first page was a form letter from the hospital CEO. Hiding my smirk, I looked at it, not believing they were actually asking us for our documented opinions on this place. I half-wondered if they chucked them straight into the trash.

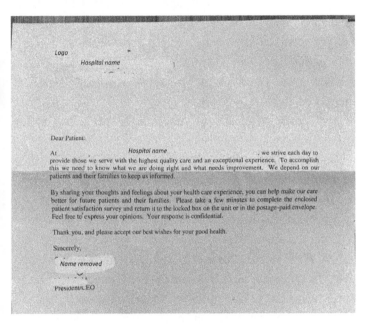

Logo

Hospital name

Dear Patient:

At *Hospital name* , we strive each day to provide those we serve with the highest quality care and an exceptional experience. To accomplish this we need to know what we are doing right and what needs improvement. We depend on our patients and their families to keep us informed.

By sharing your thoughts and feelings about your health care experience, you can help make our care better for future patients and their families. Please take a few minutes to complete the enclosed patient satisfaction survey and return it to the locked box on the unit or in the postage-paid envelope. Feel free to express your opinions. Your response is confidential.

Thank you, and please accept our best wishes for your good health.

Sincerely,

Name removed

President/CEO

"I'll need a pen," I told Liz.

"Oh, duh. Be right back."

She slipped back into the nurse's station, and I sat against the wall again to have a closer look at this survey.

The first page was a letter from the president of the hospital, saying he hoped I, the patient, had experienced the healing and therapeutic service that he and his organization were committed to delivering. I felt Mia slide down the wall next to me with her two envelopes in hand.

"Everything okay?" I asked.

"Fine. Remember how I said I'm going to that other outpatient place today? They're trying to get them on the phone to verify my treatment plan."

"Ah," I said. "But not red tape, I hope. More like yellow caution tape?"

"Probably."

"You'll still be able to leave right now though, yeah?"

Mia nodded. "That's what Mackenzie said. Just have to get them on the phone."

"Well in the meantime," I said, bringing the survey to her attention, "get a kick out of this."

Mia's eyes roamed down the page at the typed words, where questions like "Do you feel you received quality and personalized treatment during your stay?" and "Would you recommend this hospital to others?" made her eyes grow larger and larger.

"Oh, fuck yeah," she whispered. I handed her the pen that Liz had given me ("Just make sure I get it back!") and watched her crack her knuckles, ready to tell them in vivid detail about her experience and how she would *not* be returning for anything, not even a flu shot.

"Do you remember the name of that Greek myth," I asked Mia as she penned away furiously, "about the guy who goes to the Underworld to retrieve his true love from Hades. And he's told that he can bring her back to the world, but he has to trust she's behind him, because if he looks back, he'll lose her forever?"

"Orpheus and Eurydice," Mia answered absentmindedly.

"That's the one." I smiled at the comments I could discern from reading Mia's survey responses over her shoulder. She was not holding back. "Anyway," I continued. "I can promise you, when I step out these doors, I won't be looking back. Otherwise it could suck me back in."

"Mhmm," Mia muttered. "What do you think of this?" She pointed at a paragraph of her survey.

"Not even a hyperbole. Quite accurate, actually."

I finished my survey before Mia and asked Calvin to open the contraband closet for me again so I could retrieve my phone—it was still dead; the outlet was not working. By the time I returned, Mia was standing and rereading her answers. With straight faces, we handed Liz our completed surveys. She thanked us cheerily and handed me a clipboard.

"Discharge papers," she said. "Just read and sign."

There was a lot of text, but it seemed like it was just this signature between me and the doors. I pretended to scan the paragraphs and signed.

"What about me?" Mia asked as I handed the clipboard back to Liz.

Liz craned her neck to make eye contact with another nurse inside their room who shook her head. "Sorry," Liz apologized. "We're trying to get that other place on the phone still." Liz walked back into the nurse's station to file our surveys and my discharge papers. Mia and I looked at each other, realizing we were both alone in the hallway.

"What now?" I asked.

"Beats me." Mia tapped on the window. "Hello? You didn't tell us what else to do." Turning to me, she added, "The level of inconsideration in this place is fucking baffling."

Liz pointed at Calvin and we rounded upon him.

"Uh," he hesitated. "Sounds like she's good to leave," he said, pointing the end of his pen at me. "And you," he said to Mia, "need to wait until you can sign out."

"It's fine," Mia said to me before I had even opened my mouth. "Get out of here. Can you tell my boyfriend that I'll be right down? He should be downstairs."

"Are you sure you don't want me to wait?" I asked.

"Save yourself."

It did not feel right, but I had no power to influence Mia's final situation. I gave her a massive hug, gathered my things and walked toward the ward door behind Calvin. As he fumbled with the keys again, I looked down and saw Billie's bracelet on my wrist.

"Shit. Where's Billie? Have you seen her?"

But like she had been summoned, Billie came speed-walking down the hall.

"Oh, thank God," I exclaimed, dropping my things.

We hugged and as we did, she whispered in my ear, "Thanks for your note. I'll talk to you soon."

"I've got the numbers in my pocket," I assured her.

"It doesn't matter," she said, still hugging me. "I have a feeling I'll be getting out really soon too."

She let me go and held me at arm's length to get a good last look. I felt my heart swelling with emotion.

Calvin cleared his throat, holding the ward door open. "Ready?"

My heart was pounding a thousand beats per minute. "Ready."

I barely noticed the person sitting at the desk behind the

door as I made a beeline for the elevator's down button. I heard Calvin slam the ward door behind me, and moments later the elevator made a ding and opened. Once inside the cabin, I reached out for the elevator buttons and Billie's bracelet slid down my wrist as I pressed G. G for Ground Level. For Gladness. For Gratitude and for Good Things to Come.

The elevator began to descend, and yet it felt like I was rising. The fluorescent lighting inside the compartment glowed. I adjusted my grip on my paper bags and inhaled, feeling every molecule of oxygen bringing life to my limbs. Finally, the doors opened, and I stepped out into the light.

Afterword

So the big question—had the psych ward made me better?

It was hard to tell. In the days that followed, my behavior barely made sense. On my second day out of the ward, I listened to Jack's band perform but left before even saying hello. On the third day, I dyed my hair every color of the rainbow. On the fourth day, I met my cousins at Millenium Park and took them on a frenetic tour of Michigan Ave.

I strung together moments haphazardly like they were beads on the bracelet Billie made me, each more random and unique than the last, trying to fill every second with novelty. In my head, I considered it "reclaiming joy," which sounds much healthier than what I was really doing—distracting myself from the pain.

The psych ward had not dulled that pain. In some ways it had amplified it, in others it changed its form, and still, in others it merely gave me more examples. The lack of information and self-agency had been infuriating. The quality of care could have been considered criminal. The way some of the staff talked to us and treated us had been dehumanizing. And the lack of empathy and concern at all levels of the treatment system was distressing. So in combination, the experience had been—and I do not use this word this lightly—depressing. But I had tried to be committed because it had felt like I was going to die, and so it was better than dying.

But deep down, we know mental healthcare is so much more than just *not dying*, and mental health treatment must be redesigned to reflect that wherever it currently does not. It needs to be about empowering the sufferer to fully live and want to live and be excited to live. In that regard, this psych ward had failed.

I have talked to others with similar experiences. Someone put it this way: most hospital psychiatric wards are not set up to actually heal the mentally ill—they are meant to keep us safe and stable until we can get to somewhere and someone else that will actually do the hard healing work. In that regard, my sensation of being put "on ice" was more correct than I had realized.

And they are expensive. In a study[4] that looked at over a quarter-million mental health hospitalizations, the researchers found that billed charges were 2.5 times higher than the hospitals' reported costs to deliver care. The average cost of a 4.4 day inpatient treatment for depression was $3,616. For me, that amounts to costing a month of my rent per day. And this study was in 2006! (I have not come across any more research to suggest that the cost has decreased or become more comprehensible, though I imagine the cost now is higher and maybe even more confusing.)

In addition to being expensive, billing is nearly incomprehensible. That same study mentioned that the lack of transparency in pricing made it challenging to estimate the cost to society for a day of psychiatric hospitalization.

In other words, the post-docs could not even figure it out.

A few weeks later, I finally mustered up the courage to run the errand I had been avoiding: retrieving my bike where I had locked her up on the 606. I knew the longer I waited, the more likely it would be that I would find her completely scavenged. Sure enough, all that was left was her frame. Both wheels, the saddle, even the hazard lights, were gone.

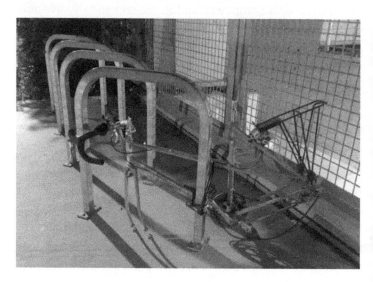

Resigned, I sat down on the same bench as before and stared out at the cars coming down Campbell street. I felt tired and sad. And lonely. My anxious fingers rubbed the wood on the bench and I looked down at clean, smooth, barely-weathered wood.

What?

They had replaced the bench. My plea for help written in permanent marker was no longer there. Some city employee, on orders of some councilman to maintain the appearance of public space, had unbolted my life raft and disposed of it someplace where things go to be disposed of, somewhere dark, odorous, full of decay. They had replaced it with a new, untarnished version, and in the process, erased the bold, blue

Sharpie evidence that I had been in crisis.

Instantly my pain felt unimportant. Everything felt suddenly impermanent and replaceable, including my life. My vision went blurry and I began to vibrate with anger and I knew I had to get off that bridge, back to my home, back to my friends.

But I only made it worse. When I arrived home I was seething, at everything and nothing, and immediately unleashed a hostile equation of angry feelings at one of my best friends. Rage had stolen the true sentence I should have said: "I am still in so much pain and I need you."

I have been open about my mental health for my entire adult life but admitting that it was still in poor condition post-hospitalization felt like cutting into my own chest. I wanted to be able to tell everyone I was okay. I was better. They had no reason to worry. I was fine. Because when I shared with people the story of the psych ward, I wanted to be able to offer a resolution to the tragedy. But the truth was that resolution would be a story in itself and that month was merely the first chapter.

My coworkers sent me flowers and I had kept them on our kitchen table as a reminder of positivity. I had seen the psychiatrist, who cut the dosage of my new Cymbalta prescription in half and apologized on behalf of her medical peers for my withdrawal experience. I eevn told my parents, one and then the other, both times crying alone in a corner after because it had felt like letting them down.

I had done what I was supposed to do—receive well wishes, see the doctor, inform my loved ones—but it had barely made a difference on how I felt.

So once more—had the psych ward made me better?

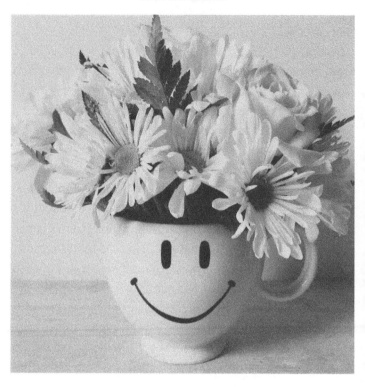

I am not convinced it was supposed to. I had hoped it would. I had gone there believing it *should.* But again, perhaps psych wards are just meant to save our lives so that, once we are out, we can continue to seek out a life worth living. (As for what makes life worth living? You can get that answer from other books.)

I think overall, the psych ward had been a disappointment. It did not make me better, and my mental, emotional, and physical health all deteriorated in varying degrees during my stay. I had entered in pain and then been discharged feeling much the same, just more coherent!

What began to make me better was the same thing as always: acknowledging that I was suffering and then, in any given moment, taking as big a step as I could to try to lessen that suffering. One day it was sitting outside on the grass, eating Miko's Italian ice with friends. Another day it was pushing past my couch-tied inertia to go to a Chicago Cub's game with coworkers. Most days it was just making sure I ate two or more meals, got fresh air, and talked to someone who cared about me.

What made me better was time. Time and reflection.

Though reflecting was a mixed bag. Writing this story was reflection. Trying to glean meaning from the experience was reflection. (Did you know they added this as a sixth stage to the 'five stages of grief'?) I wanted there to be lessons, or maybe new truths, and so I wrote some down: everybody hurts, everybody is doing their best, everybody smiles at rainbows, everybody wants to be understood.

But those were things I had learned during the entire span of my life thus far, not succinctly during my time spent on the fifteenth floor.

It is now nearly three years later. I live in Cambridge, Massachusetts. At work, I sit at a desk that I have decorated with Lego mini-figures of Wonder Woman, Black Widow, and Captain Marvel and do not care about promotions or salary or that I am mixing comic book universes. Than is engaged and we have a weekly Zoom call with our friends to play games and catch up. And though I have tried to deny it, I am deep in another valley of depression.

I am as prepared as ever though! I call my friends. I go to the gym. I get eight hours of sleep. I eat healthy meals and get enough vitamins. I remind myself of the psychology lessons about how the mind misleads us. I meditate. I journal every day. I see a therapist.

And most of all, hardest of all, I try not to look at the speed of the lives of those around me. My friends talk about having kids and I wonder if I could ever take care of children when it takes so much effort to just take care of myself. I get lonely. I get tired. I lose the ability to concentrate in the middle of the day. I get angry at myself and take it out on the ones I love. Accomplishments do not bring me joy or fulfillment. Recognition feels unearned. Food tastes bland. I am a specter at gatherings and then leave early. I am a zombie on the streets and avoid eye contact with strangers. I try, I *try*, to savor and show gratitude and appreciate the sun on my face, but none of it feels like it should.

This is depression.

It is odd. A story should follow a framework. Exposition evolves into rising action, which takes us to a narrative climax, that dissolves into falling action and ushers in the resolution. But here I was, telling you a tale while knowing full well that there would be little resolved in its end. (Maybe that's why people in their twenties should wait before they write anything akin to a memoir!) How dare I attempt to tell the story then?

Well, because that is just the reality of it, and that is okay.

There are two reasons I wrote this down and committed to letting it leave the safety of my own journal. The first reason was selfish. I knew it would help me heal. I needed the distraction (and like any woman will tell you, we excel when given a project.) I hoped sharing it would help me both connect and find better aid.

The second reason was for you, if you, like me, sometimes battle yourself to stave off sadness, and need to be reminded that you are not alone in the fight. Or if you care for someone fighting and wanted to better understand what they might be feeling.

Mental illness will never disappear. Its cousins, isolation and loneliness and anguish, will never disappear. We need allies to fight, and this story is like a petition asking you to commit to the cause. Because it does feel like a fight, like a battle, and if we approach it that way, then it does not seem so crazy to want to pore over a table and strategize. Identify the enemy—depression. Inventory the weapons—therapy, healthy habits, communities. Look for alliances—loved ones. The better the strategy and the bigger the army, the greater the odds at triumph.

So still we soldier on. Though sometimes in a uniform of sock-feet and sweatpants, we soldier on. On and on and on until tomorrow.

References

1. Hansen, Olivia. "Rice Maintains 'Happiest Students' Status by Ousting Unhappy Students." The Rice Thresher, 29 Nov. 2012, web.archive.org/web/20121214225343 /www.ricethresher.org/rice-maintains-happiest-students-status-by-ousting-unhappy-students-1.2961393.

2. Kingkade, Tyler. "Using College Mental Health Services Can Lead To Students Getting Removed From Campus." *The Huffington Post*, 7 Dec. 2017, www.huffingtonpost.com/2014/10/07/college-mental-health-services_n_5900632.html.

3. Schwartz, Victor. "Mandatory Leave of Absence for College Students With Suicidal Behaviors: The Real Story." *Psychiatric Times*, 26 Aug. 2016, www.psychiatrictimes.com/suicide/mandatory-leave-absence-college-students-suicidal-behaviors-real-story.

4. Stensland, Michael, et al. "An Examination of Costs, Charges, and Payments for Inpatient Psychiatric Treatment in Community Hospitals." *Psychiatric Services (Washington, D.C.)*, U.S. National Library of Medicine, July 2012, www.ncbi.nlm.nih.gov/pubmed/22588167.

You are never alone.

National Suicide Prevention Lifeline:
1-800-273-8255